CW01455312

The N A F L D Mastery Bible: Your Blueprint For Complete N A F L D Management

Dr. Ankita Kashyap and Prof. Krishna N. Sharma

Published by Virtued Press, 2023.

While every precaution has been taken in the preparation of this book, the publisher assumes no responsibility for errors or omissions, or for damages resulting from the use of the information contained herein.

THE N A F L D MASTERY BIBLE: YOUR BLUEPRINT FOR COMPLETE N A F L D MANAGEMENT

First edition. November 20, 2023.

ISBN: 979-8223065319

Written by Dr. Ankita Kashyap and Prof. Krishna N. Sharma.

Table of Contents

DISCLAIMER

The information provided in this book is intended for general informational purposes only. The content is not meant to substitute professional medical advice, diagnosis, or treatment. Always consult with a qualified healthcare provider before making any changes to your diabetes management plan or healthcare regimen.

While every effort has been made to ensure the accuracy and completeness of the information presented, the author and publisher do not assume any responsibility for errors, omissions, or potential misinterpretations of the content. Individual responses to diabetes management strategies may vary, and what works for one person might not be suitable for another.

The book does not endorse any specific medical treatments, products, or services. Readers are encouraged to seek guidance from their healthcare providers to determine the most appropriate approaches for their unique medical conditions and needs.

Any external links or resources provided in the book are for convenience and informational purposes only. The author and publisher do not have control over the content or availability of these external sources and do not endorse or guarantee the accuracy of such information.

Readers are advised to exercise caution and use their judgment when applying the information provided in this book to their own situations. The author and publisher disclaim any liability for any direct, indirect, consequential, or other damages arising from the use of this book and its content.

By reading and using this book, readers acknowledge and accept the limitations and inherent risks associated with implementing the strategies, recommendations, and information contained herein. It is always recommended to consult a qualified healthcare professional for personalized medical advice and care.

Chapter 7: Conclusion

Introduction

Have you ever pondered what it might be like to live with a secret inside of you? An unseen hazard that never raises any red flags and endangers your pleasure and well-being? Now, my dear readers, allow me to take you on a voyage into the mysterious depths of non-alcoholic fatty liver disease, or NAFLD, where change and mastery are waiting to be discovered.

I'm sitting here with a pen in hand and a piece of parchment in front of me, and I'm fascinated by how intricate the human body is. Every note played in this exquisite symphony, this work of art in motion, influences the overall harmony. And the liver is the main character in this symphony. The liver, oh! A secret organ, mostly ignored until its whispers become cries, silently humming in the shadows and performing its essential activities.

Fatty Liver Disease Without Alcohol Use. The very mention of the name piques my curiosity. Because it is not an illness brought on by overindulgence, but rather a silent invader that can affect even the most morally upright people. Though misdiagnosed and misunderstood by many, this ailment nonetheless casts a shadow over countless lives at night.

Now, let's set out on this adventure together, dear reader. Let's explore the complexities of non-alcoholic fatty liver disease and uncover its mysteries. I have painstakingly stitched together knowledge strands in this holy book, pulling from the wisdom of holistic health techniques as well as the fabric of medical science. My goal is to close the gap between the clinical and the humane, the scientific and the spiritual, through my writing.

In my capacity as a physician and health and wellness advisor, I have committed my practise to assisting patients affected by this silent threat. We have worked to reduce the pain and rekindle hope with my team of professionals from a range of wellness and health-related

3

sectors. However, simply treating the symptoms and bandaging the wound is insufficient. No, reader, we have to go a little further.

You will discover a wealth of knowledge within the pages, with every word selected with care to give you power. I have read through reputable medical journals, sifted through reputable scientific papers, and developed a fact-based route. However, I promise not to burden you with intimidating language or unintelligible prose. No, my pen moves smoothly over the page, leaving clear, crisp phrases in its wake for you to comprehend with each stroke.

I give you more than just a passing glance into the realm of NAFLD in this book. I offer you a road map, a beacon of light to help you through the maze-like passageways of this illness. I am your friend, your confidante, and your mentor as soon as you turn the pages of these pages. We are going to go on a transformational and therapeutic journey together.

I am aware that every reader is different and has a unique tale to share. For this reason, I have created individualised programmes and self-help methods that can change as your life does. Although every trip is unique, you will discover the resources you need on these pages to revive your energy and change the course of your life.

I beg you, my dear reader, to read these words as a balm for your tired spirit rather than just as ink on paper. Allow my fanciful prose and mellow tone to surround you like a warm, loving hug. Let the words tickle your senses, like a cool summer's day breeze whispering through the foliage. We will set out on a path of healing and exploration together, one that will bring about transformation and the blossoming of knowledge.

So come along with me, reader, as we unravel the mysteries behind non-alcoholic fatty liver disease. Let's embrace the enigma, the skill, and the boundless potential that are all inside of us. We will emerge from the shadows as a team and pave the way for total NAFLD control.

Allow this holy book to serve as your refuge, your guide, and your model for a transformed life.

Chapter 1: A Comprehensive Guide

Understanding Non Alcoholic Fatty Liver Disease

It is crucial to examine the meaning and context of NAFLD in order to fully comprehend it. The condition known as non-alcoholic fatty liver disease is defined by an excessive buildup of fat in the liver in people who drink little or no alcohol. Steatosis—excess fat—infiltrates the liver cells and can result in inflammation and scarring. This can set the stage for more serious disorders like cirrhosis, fibrosis, non-alcoholic steatohepatitis (NASH), and even liver failure. In the world today, NAFLD is thought to be the most prevalent kind of chronic liver disease.

What then are NAFLD's causes? Research suggests that there are multiple contributing elements, even though the precise explanation is still not entirely understood. Obesity—more specifically, extra fat accumulated in the abdomen region or abdominal obesity—is the main risk factor. Insulin resistance, metabolic syndrome, type 2 diabetes, elevated blood pressure, elevated cholesterol, and a sedentary lifestyle are additional factors that may heighten the likelihood of developing non-alcoholic fatty liver disease (NAFLD).

Many people with NAFLD may not have any symptoms at all, and the disease's symptoms can vary greatly. For the purpose of early detection, this emphasises how important it is to have routine health check-ups and tests. When symptoms do occur, they are common and include weakness, exhaustion, and abdominal pain. In more severe cases, they can also include jaundice, which is a yellowing of the skin and eyes, swelling in the legs and abdomen, and mental confusion.

Addressing the risk factors and taking proactive measures for prevention and management are crucial given the possible consequences that untreated NAFLD may cause. One of the most important aspects of managing NAFLD is changing one's lifestyle.

Changes in eating patterns, more exercise, weight loss, and treating underlying medical issues like diabetes and high blood pressure are a few examples of these adjustments.

A well-balanced diet is essential when making dietary adjustments. Limiting intake of meals high in added sugars and saturated fats, as well as processed and fried foods, is crucial. Eat a range of fruits, vegetables, whole grains, lean meats, and healthy fats like avocados, nuts, and seeds as an alternative. Including particular foods, such as green tea, coffee, turmeric, garlic, and cruciferous vegetables like broccoli and Brussels sprouts, that have been demonstrated to boost liver health can also be advantageous.

To enhance liver health and general well-being, frequent physical exercise is crucial in addition to dietary modifications. Aerobic exercise can help lower body fat and increase insulin sensitivity. Examples of this type of exercise include jogging, cycling, and brisk walking. Exercises involving strength training, like weightlifting or resistance band workouts, can also help with muscle growth and metabolic enhancement. Try to complete two or more days of strength training and at least 150 minutes of moderate- to vigorous-intense aerobic activity or 75 minutes of intense aerobic activity per week.

It is significant to emphasise that a comprehensive strategy is needed to manage NAFLD. Addressing underlying psychological and emotional causes is critical in addition to lifestyle improvements. Stress, poor self-esteem, and body image problems are common among NAFLD patients, and these conditions can hinder their capacity to make life-improving decisions. I work directly with my patients as a health and wellness coach, offering them coping mechanisms, self-help tactics, psychology-related skills, and counselling to support them on their path to better liver health.

A thorough approach for managing non-alcoholic fatty liver disease can also incorporate complementary and alternative techniques. These could involve techniques like mindfulness, yoga, acupuncture, and meditation, which have been demonstrated to improve general wellbeing, lower stress levels, and support liver health.

In conclusion, multifaceted therapy is necessary for the optimal treatment of nonalcoholic fatty liver disease, which is a difficult disorder. People can take proactive measures for liver health improvement and prevention by being aware of the causes, symptoms, and risk factors of nonalcoholic fatty liver disease (NAFLD). People can take back control of their health and stop NAFLD from worsening into more serious liver diseases by making lifestyle changes, such as eating different foods, exercising more, and treating psychological and emotional issues. People can achieve full NAFLD control and optimal well-being by adopting a holistic strategy that takes into account their mind, body, and spirit.

The Importance of Management

The disorder known as nonalcoholic fatty liver disease (NAFLD) is brought on by an abnormal buildup of fat in the liver in people who drink little to no alcohol. Research indicates that it affects about 25% of the world's population, and that it is getting more common in contemporary society (Younossi et al., 2019). Neglecting the treatment of non-alcoholic fatty liver disease (NAFLD) can result in the development of more serious liver disorders, including cirrhosis, non-alcoholic steatohepatitis (NASH), and even liver cancer, even though it may frequently go undetected in its early stages (Musso et al., 2019). These possible outcomes emphasise how urgently NAFLD care is required.

The fact that NAFLD is silent in the early stages is one of the reasons it is frequently ignored. Until the disease has proceeded to a more severe level, many people might not even be aware that they have it. For this reason, routine screenings and examinations are crucial to early identification and treatment. People with nonalcoholic fatty liver disease (NAFLD) can stop or slow the condition's progression to more serious liver illnesses.

Neglecting to control non-alcoholic fatty liver disease (NAFLD) can also have a negative effect on general health and wellbeing. According to research, people with non-alcoholic fatty liver disease (NAFLD) have an increased likelihood of developing other chronic illnesses, including metabolic syndrome, type 2 diabetes, and cardiovascular disease (Younossi et al., 2019). These illnesses have the potential to aggravate the course of NAFLD and make care even more difficult. People can lower their chance of acquiring these related disorders and enhance their general health outcomes by managing their NAFLD proactively.

Additionally, one's quality of life may suffer significantly if NAFLD is not managed. People may develop symptoms including weariness, jaundice, and abdominal pain as the illness worsens, which can have a significant impact on their everyday activities and general health. Furthermore, NAFLD may result in problems such liver cirrhosis, which can impair liver function and necessitate liver transplantation. In addition to their bodily effects, these repercussions may lead to financial hardship and psychological anguish for the affected individuals and their family. People with non-alcoholic fatty liver disease (NAFLD) can enhance their quality of life and lessen the disease's negative effects on their general health by actively controlling it.

It's crucial to remember that managing NAFLD entails more than just addressing the illness's outward manifestations. Numerous environmental and lifestyle factors might have an impact on this illness, which is frequently complex in nature. Therefore, in order to address every component of the condition, a holistic approach to management is required. Making lifestyle changes, such as switching to a nutritious diet, exercising frequently, controlling stress, and getting enough sleep, is part of this. Counseling and psychological approaches can also be helpful in addressing the mental and emotional elements of NAFLD. People can control NAFLD and lessen its possible effects by implementing a thorough management plan that includes all of these elements.

In summary, it is critical to take proactive measures to manage nonalcoholic fatty liver disease. Ignoring this illness increases the chance of acquiring other chronic ailments and can cause more serious liver diseases to progress. It may also negatively affect a person's general wellbeing and quality of life. People can improve their overall health outcomes and stop or slow the advancement of NAFLD by managing their condition pro-actively. In order to give NAFLD management top priority and advance holistic healthcare and wellness, it is critical to comprehend the possible repercussions of disregarding the condition.

How This Book Can Help You

The purpose of this extensive book is to describe the various ways in which it might offer useful knowledge and management techniques for nonalcoholic fatty liver disease. Through a methodical approach, this book seeks to provide you the tools to take charge of your health and well-being, guiding you through the intricacies of this condition and helping you reach the best possible state of liver health.

1. Understanding Non Alcoholic Fatty Liver Disease

Understanding the condition itself is the first step towards effective management. In order to shed light on the causes, risk factors, symptoms, and course of non-alcoholic fatty liver disease, I go further into its complexities in this book. I give a succinct and straightforward explanation of how this condition impacts your liver and general health, based on the most recent research and medical knowledge.

2. Identifying Personal Risk Factors

In your particular case, it is critical to determine the precise risk factors that contribute to the onset and progression of nonalcoholic fatty liver disease. Through a thorough evaluation that looks at your lifestyle, genetic predispositions, and medical history, I help you identify the variables that could be making your disease worse. With this knowledge at your disposal, you will be more qualified to create a management strategy that works.

3. Lifestyle Modifications

Adopting substantial lifestyle changes is necessary for the management of non-alcoholic fatty liver disease. I go over the main areas in this book where you may make significant adjustments to improve the health of your liver. I offer a comprehensive approach to changing your lifestyle for the better, encompassing everything from nutritional changes to exercise regimens, stress management tactics, sleep hygiene practises, and smoking cessation measures. I stress how important it is to design a sustainable plan that works for your unique circumstances and tastes so that you may make long-lasting changes.

4. Personalized Food and Diet Planning

Nutrition is a key component of the management of nonalcoholic fatty liver disease. Food is essential for maintaining liver health and counteracting the illness's consequences. I work with qualified nutritionists to assist you in developing a customised food and diet plan that meets your specific requirements. This entails knowing which foods are good for the liver, controlling portion sizes, and creating scrumptious yet nourishing meal plans. You can enhance general wellness and maximise liver function by consuming the proper ratio of nutrients.

5. Counselling and Psychology-Related Techniques

Managing a chronic illness like nonalcoholic fatty liver disease can be detrimental to your mental and emotional well-being. To attain holistic wellbeing, it is imperative to address the psychological aspects of managing this illness. I introduce you to the power of psychology-related procedures and therapy within the pages of this book. You will discover evidence-based methods for stress management, overcoming negative thought patterns, building resilience, and encouraging constructive lifestyle adjustments. You can effectively manage your disease by taking good care of your mental and emotional health.

6. Self-Care Alternative and Complementary Techniques

This book examines complementary and alternative forms of self-care in addition to conventional medical methods. I firmly believe in the efficacy of holistic therapies, which include yoga, meditation, acupuncture, herbal cures, and other holistic activities. Through the integration of these traditional methods with the finest aspects of Western medicine, we can enhance the effectiveness of our management techniques by harnessing the body's innate healing capacity. This book acts as a roadmap to assist you in investigating and incorporating these methods into your individual path toward liver health.

7. Self-Help Techniques and Coping Strategies

It can be difficult to manage nonalcoholic fatty liver disease on both a physical and mental level. I offer a wide range of self-help methods and coping skills to help you get over these challenges. These include ways to deal with pain, ways to deal with exhaustion, ways to increase the quality of your sleep, and ways to make your life better overall. You can manage this condition with confidence and elegance by arming yourself with these tools and methods, which will help you through its ups and downs.

"The Non Alcoholic Fatty Liver Disease Mastery Bible: Your Blueprint for Complete Non Alcoholic Fatty Liver Disease Management" is a book that, in essence, attempts to provide you the tools you need to take control of your health and fitness. This book offers specific strategies for managing non-alcoholic fatty liver disease through a step-by-step guide. These strategies include understanding the condition, identifying personal risk factors, changing lifestyle choices, developing individualised food and diet plans, embracing counselling and psychology-related techniques, investigating alternative and complementary self-care techniques, and arming yourself with coping mechanisms and self-help techniques. I cordially encourage you to set out on this path to the best possible liver health and a happy life.

Chapter 2: Understanding the Liver

Liver Anatomy and Physiology

The largest glandular organ in the body is the liver, which is situated in the upper right side of the abdomen. It is separated into two main lobes, the left and right lobes, and weighs about three pounds. These lobes can be further subdivided into lobules, which are smaller lobes.

Each lobule is made up of individual liver cells grouped in a distinct pattern at the microscopic level. These cells specialise in different aspects of metabolism and detoxification. Blood veins such as the hepatic artery and the portal vein, which supply oxygenated and nutrient-rich blood, respectively, are abundant in the liver.

With over 500 distinct bodily activities, the liver is a true multitasking organ. Let's examine a few of its main purposes:

1. Metabolism: The process of metabolism, which includes converting lipids, proteins, and carbs into forms that may be used, is carried out by the liver. By either releasing stored glycogen as needed or converting excess glucose to glycogen for storage, it controls blood glucose levels. It is also essential for the synthesis of new proteins and the breakdown of existing ones in the process of protein metabolism.

2. Bile Production: Bile is a fluid that is produced by the liver and is crucial for digestion. Bile salts, which are found in bile, help the small intestine break down and absorb fats. Additionally, it aids in the body's removal of waste products like bilirubin, which is produced when red blood cells break down.

3. Detoxification: Detoxification is a vital part of the liver's job. It removes poisons, alcohol, and other dangerous compounds from the blood. The body then transforms these compounds into less toxic forms and excretes them.

4. Storage: A variety of minerals and vitamins are stored in the liver. Together with iron and copper, it stores the vitamins A, D, E, and K. It also stores glycogen, which when needed for energy, can be converted into glucose.

5. Immune Function: Due to its ability to produce immunological components and eliminate toxins and pathogens from the bloodstream, the liver is an essential component of the body's immune system. It also aids in the synthesis of factors that coagulate blood.

It is essential to comprehend the anatomy and physiology of the liver in order to effectively manage non-alcoholic fatty liver disease. This disorder develops when too much fat builds up in the liver cells, which can cause inflammation and even damage to the liver. Understanding the complex functions of the liver allows us to create efficient plans for both prevention and treatment.

The care of non-alcoholic fatty liver disease necessitates a strong emphasis on lifestyle changes, including eating a nutritious diet and exercising frequently. The amount of fat that builds up in the liver can be decreased with a balanced diet high in fruits, vegetables, whole grains, and low in processed foods, refined sugars, and saturated fats.

Frequent exercise can help manage non-alcoholic fatty liver disease by promoting weight loss and improving insulin sensitivity. For at least 150 minutes a week, performing cardiovascular workouts, such swimming or brisk walking, can significantly improve liver health.

Techniques from psychology and counselling are also useful in the treatment of non-alcoholic fatty liver disease. It is important to recognise the emotional and psychological toll that this illness can have. Feelings of anxiety, annoyance, and guilt are possible for patients. Through psychological approaches and therapy, we can assist people in creating coping mechanisms to deal with the difficulties of managing this illness.

The management of non-alcoholic fatty liver disease might include a variety of alternative and complementary self-care strategies in addition to lifestyle adjustments and counselling. These methods could include herbal remedies, yoga, acupuncture, and meditation. Although further studies are necessary to completely comprehend the efficacy of these methods, they have demonstrated potential in promoting liver function and general wellbeing.

It is crucial to handle non-alcoholic fatty liver disease holistically. We can customise therapy regimens to target the underlying causes of the illness and support long-term liver health by taking into account the structure and physiology of the liver. When it comes to giving people with non-alcoholic fatty liver disease full treatment and support, working together with a team of professionals from many health and wellness sectors is essential.

I am dedicated to assisting my patients in achieving maximum liver health as a medical doctor and health and wellness coach by way of lifestyle changes, counselling, self-care practises, and teamwork. By working together, we can enable people to successfully manage non-alcoholic fatty liver disease and regain control over their health.

Recall that the liver is an amazing organ with tremendous regenerating powers. We can improve our quality of life by restoring the health and vitality of our liver through healthy lifestyle modifications.

Liver Health and Non Alcoholic Fatty Liver Disease

It's crucial to have a fundamental understanding of the liver in order to fully comprehend how NAFLD affects liver health. The liver is an amazing organ that is essential to the general operation of our body. It is in charge of detoxifying dangerous compounds, generating bile to aid in digestion, storing vitamins and minerals, controlling blood sugar, and creating the blood-clotting proteins.

When we discuss nonalcoholic fatty liver disease (NAFLD), we are referring to a condition where the liver has an excessive accumulation of fat. This disorder can vary from non-alcoholic steatohepatitis (NASH), which causes inflammation and damage to the liver cells, to simple fatty liver, which is limited to fat buildup in the liver. If NAFLD is not treated, it can lead to more serious diseases such liver cancer, cirrhosis, and liver failure.

How therefore does liver health relate to NAFLD? The buildup of fat is one of the main alterations that take place in the liver. The liver typically contains a minor quantity of fat. Nonetheless, there is an aberrant accumulation of fat within the liver cells in those who have NAFLD. One condition that may result from this fat accumulation is hepatosteatosis. Hepatosteatosis can affect the liver's essential processes, including bile generation and detoxification, which can make it more difficult for the liver to operate normally.

NAFLD causes inflammation in the liver in addition to fat storage. When our body's immune system perceives the excess fat in the liver as a danger, it launches an attack on the liver cells, resulting in inflammation. This immune reaction has the potential to harm liver cells, leading to scarring and death of the liver cells. This scarring has the potential to develop into cirrhosis over time, which is a disorder marked by severe liver fibrosis and decreased liver function.

Moreover, NAFLD throws off the balance of liver enzymes, which are in charge of the liver's synthesis and breakdown of a variety of substances. People with non-alcoholic fatty liver disease (NAFLD) frequently have elevated levels of liver enzymes, including alanine aminotransferase (ALT) and aspartate aminotransferase (AST). When there is damage to the liver cells, these enzymes are released into the bloodstream. The diagnosis and tracking of NAFLD can be aided by keeping an eye on the levels of these enzymes.

Additionally, NAFLD and metabolic syndrome are linked to insulin resistance. When our cells lose their sensitivity to the hormone insulin, which controls blood sugar levels, we develop insulin resistance. Insulin resistance has the potential to cause the liver to produce more glucose, which would raise blood sugar levels. Conversely, metabolic syndrome is a collection of disorders that includes insulin resistance, high blood pressure, obesity, and high cholesterol. The onset and course of non-alcoholic fatty liver disease are intimately associated with both insulin resistance and metabolic syndrome.

In conclusion, NAFLD is a multifaceted illness that has an impact on liver health in various ways. Hepatosteatosis, a condition caused by the accumulation of fat in the liver, compromises the liver's normal functioning. NAFLD-related inflammation can harm and scar liver cells, which can result in more severe diseases like cirrhosis. The detrimental effects of NAFLD on liver health are further compounded by the disturbance of liver enzymes and the correlation with insulin resistance and metabolic syndrome.

It is critical to address the underlying causes of NAFLD and make the required lifestyle alterations in order to effectively treat the condition and enhance liver function. This can entail giving up processed meals, sugar-filled drinks, and binge drinking in favour of a balanced diet high in fruits, vegetables, whole grains, lean meats, and healthy fats. Maintaining a healthy weight, practising stress management, and engaging in regular physical activity can all significantly enhance liver function.

Depending on how severe NAFLD is, medical measures could also be required in addition to lifestyle changes. These could include drugs to treat underlying illnesses like diabetes, hypertension, and elevated cholesterol. Additionally, regular blood testing and imaging examinations can help closely monitor liver function, which can help guide treatment decisions and assess the course of nonalcoholic fatty liver disease.

I'm dedicated to assisting people with non-alcoholic fatty liver disease (NAFLD) in taking control of their health and managing their illness holistically as a health and wellness coach. Not only may NAFLD be managed, but liver health and general well-being can be enhanced by addressing lifestyle issues, encouraging good habits, and collaborating with a team of experts from other health and wellness sectors. Individuals can genuinely take charge of their non-alcoholic fatty liver disease and make progress toward a better future if they have the necessary information, encouragement, and commitment.

I hope this chapter clarified the unique alterations that NAFLD causes in the liver and underlined the significance of being proactive in maintaining liver health. To further our comprehension of this intricate ailment, we will explore the risk factors and causes of NAFLD in greater detail in the upcoming chapter.

Risk Factors for Non Alcoholic Fatty Liver Disease

One important risk factor for NAFLD is obesity, which is sometimes referred to as the silent epidemic of the twenty-first century. I have direct experience with the negative effects of obesity on an individual's general health as a medical practitioner and health and wellness coach, with NAFLD being one of the most prevalent side effects. Obesity and nonalcoholic fatty liver disease (NAFLD) have a complex relationship, with the primary pathological characteristic being an abnormal buildup of fat in the liver.

Why is there a higher chance of NAFLD among obese people? Well, being overweight sets off a series of metabolic alterations that are ideal for the emergence of non-alcoholic fatty liver disease (NAFLD). Obese people's adipose tissue releases more free fatty acids into the bloodstream, where the liver absorbs them. The overabundance of fatty acids surpasses the liver's ability to process them, causing fat droplets to accumulate in the hepatocytes, or liver cells.

Furthermore, obesity accelerates the course of non-alcoholic fatty liver disease (NAFLD) by causing a condition of persistent low-grade inflammation. Cytokines, which are chemicals that cause inflammation, are secreted by adipose tissue and have the ability to enter the liver and cause inflammation. This inflammation encourages damage to the liver and the growth of fibrosis, which can lead to cirrhosis and even liver cancer if untreated.

Let's now examine the strong connection between NAFLD and diabetes. Diabetes is thought to be a significant risk factor for NAFLD, particularly type 2 diabetes. Actually, studies have indicated that NAFLD coexists with type 2 diabetes in as many as 70% of cases. These two illnesses are related by the metabolic problems they share, such as dysregulated lipid metabolism and insulin resistance.

Insulin resistance, a defining feature of type 2 diabetes and prediabetes, is typified by a reduction in the body's sensitivity to insulin, the hormone that controls blood sugar levels. In order to make up for this, the pancreas generates more insulin, which in turn encourages the liver to manufacture more fat. NAFLD results from the liver's inability to remove fat from the bloodstream due to excessive fat synthesis.

Moreover, another important factor contributing to the development of NAFLD in diabetics is dysregulated lipid metabolism. Increased triglyceride and low-density lipoprotein (LDL) levels are linked to the build-up of hepatic fat. Diabetes is frequently associated with these excessive lipid levels because of metabolic abnormalities such high blood glucose and poor lipid breakdown.

Although diabetes and obesity are well-known risk factors for nonalcoholic fatty liver disease (NAFLD), it is important to take specific drugs' effects on liver health into account. Both prescription and over-the-counter medications have the potential to cause liver damage, a condition known as hepatotoxic consequences. Certain drugs worsen pre-existing liver damage, while others are directly linked to the development of NAFLD.

The drug class typically associated with non-alcoholic fatty liver disease (NAFLD) includes corticosteroids, or steroids. These potent anti-inflammatory medications are used for a number of ailments, such as asthma, autoimmune illnesses, and some forms of cancer. Nevertheless, because corticosteroids can worsen liver inflammation and fat deposition, prolonged or high-dose usage of these drugs has been connected to the onset of nonalcoholic fatty liver disease (NAFLD).

Certain antiviral medicine types used for HIV treatment are another class of pharmaceuticals that may cause non-alcoholic fatty liver disease (NAFLD). These medications, sometimes referred to as nucleoside reverse transcriptase inhibitors, or NRTIs, have been linked to a higher risk of NAFLD and other liver-related issues. While receiving antiviral medication, it's critical for people with HIV to collaborate closely with their doctor to check the state of their liver.

It's crucial to remember that excessive alcohol usage can greatly raise the chance of having NAFLD in addition to these particular drugs. Although alcoholic liver disease and nonalcoholic fatty liver disease are different conditions, they can coexist and worsen each other's effects on the liver. Therefore, it is essential to entirely refrain from alcohol consumption for those who have NAFLD in order to stop additional liver damage.

To sum up, in order to effectively manage and prevent this increasingly common liver disease, it is imperative to recognise the risk factors for nonalcoholic fatty liver disease (NAFLD). Risks associated with diabetes, obesity, and some drugs must be managed with appropriate medical therapies, vigilant monitoring, and lifestyle changes. As a physician and health and wellness coach, I implore you to take charge of your health by identifying these risk factors and pursuing a thorough management strategy for nonalcoholic fatty liver disease.

Liver Function Tests

Prior to delving into the particulars of liver function tests, it's critical to comprehend the liver's critical function in our general health. The liver is an amazing organ that performs many vital tasks for the body, such as storing vitamins and minerals, regulating blood sugar levels, detoxifying toxic substances, generating bile to aid with digestion, and manufacturing proteins, cholesterol, and clotting factors.

The purpose of the liver function tests is to evaluate the liver's ability to function, spot any anomalies, and help diagnose liver illnesses, such as NAFLD. Analyzing patient-supplied blood samples is typically part of these examinations. It's crucial to remember that while these tests are not NAFLD-specific, they can offer insightful information about liver health.

1. Alanine Aminotransferase (ALT):

The liver is the primary location for the enzyme ALT, and elevated levels of this enzyme in the blood can suggest inflammation or damage to the liver. Often, the first warning sign of liver damage is elevated ALT levels. Increased fat buildup in the liver in NAFLD patients might result in inflammation and raised ALT levels. On the other hand, hepatitis caused by viruses and liver damage brought on by drugs can also cause increased ALT levels. Interpreting ALT results in light of other liver function tests and clinical assessment is therefore essential.

2. Aspartate Aminotransferase (AST):

Another enzyme, called AST, is mostly located in the liver but is also found in the heart and muscles. Similar to ALT, increased AST values indicate inflammation or injury to the liver. But in contrast to ALT, AST levels are also subject to external influences. For instance, cardiac conditions or muscular damage can potentially cause an increase in AST levels. To obtain a more accurate assessment of liver health, it is crucial to interpret AST results in conjunction with other liver function tests and clinical observations.

3. Alkaline Phosphatase (ALP):

During pregnancy, the enzyme ALP is present in the placenta, bones, and intestines in addition to the liver. Increased ALP readings may indicate bone or liver disorders. Elevated ALP levels in NAFLD may be linked to cholestasis, a disorder in which the liver's ability to excrete bile is compromised, and liver inflammation. Tracking changes in ALP levels over time can be useful in determining how the liver disease is progressing or getting better.

4. Gamma-Glutamyl Transferase (GGT):

The hepatic and biliary systems are the primary locations for GGT. A common finding in liver disorders, such as NAFLD, is elevated GGT levels. It's crucial to rule out alcohol-related liver illness when interpreting GGT data because alcohol usage can potentially raise GGT levels. An blockage of the bile flow or liver disease may also be indicated by elevated GGT levels.

5. Total Bilirubin:

One yellow pigment created during the destruction of red blood cells is called bilirubin. The combined amount of conjugated and unconjugated bilirubin is known as total bilirubin. A liver disease or impaired liver function may be indicated by elevated total bilirubin levels. Unless there is an underlying liver lesion or other issues, bilirubin levels in NAFLD are typically within the normal range.

6. Serum Albumin:

The liver produces albumin, a protein that is essential for both transferring different chemicals and preserving blood osmotic pressure. Due to insufficient albumin production by the liver, low blood albumin levels may be a sign of poor liver function. It's crucial to remember that other conditions like malnutrition or renal illness can also result in lower albumin levels. As a result, it's important to consider additional liver function tests and clinical evaluation when interpreting serum albumin levels.

7. Prothrombin Time (PT) and International Normalized Ratio (INR):

The prothrombin time is a measurement of the blood clotting time. It is employed to evaluate how well the liver produces clotting factors. Impaired liver function may be indicated by an elevated PT or INR. PT or INR levels in NAFLD are often within normal limits unless cirrhosis or severe liver impairment are present.

Other tests may be conducted in addition to these widely used liver function tests in order to assess the severity of NAFLD, further evaluate liver functioning, and rule out other liver illnesses. Hepatitis B and C screening, liver biopsy, FibroScan, liver ultrasound, and imaging tests like magnetic resonance elastography are a few examples of these examinations (MRE).

Interpreting liver function tests in conjunction with other clinical findings and imaging examinations is essential to appropriately identify nonalcoholic fatty liver disease (NAFLD) and determine the degree of liver damage. Keep in mind that liver function tests are only one component of the puzzle, and that managing NAFLD holistically requires a comprehensive strategy.

We will explore a variety of dietary strategies, lifestyle adjustments, and supportive tactics in the upcoming chapter to assist effectively manage nonalcoholic fatty liver disease (NAFLD). In order to treat the underlying causes of NAFLD and enhance liver health, which will ultimately improve general well-being, a comprehensive approach to the disease's care is needed. Follow along as we uncover additional secrets and tactics in our quest to conquer nonalcoholic fatty liver disease.

Liver-Related Complications

Cirrhosis is one of the possible side effects of nonalcoholic fatty liver disease. The normal liver tissue is replaced by scar tissue in cirrhosis, a late stage of liver disease that impairs the liver's normal functioning. It gets more difficult for the liver to perform essential tasks like removing toxins from the blood, making bile, and storing vitamins and minerals as it is scarred. Numerous problems and symptoms follow from this.

A person's general health can be significantly impacted by the dangerous illness known as cirrhosis. It might result in symptoms like weight loss, exhaustion, jaundice, and itching. Furthermore, problems including ascites (a accumulation of fluid in the abdomen), hepatic encephalopathy (a disorder that affects brain function), and varices are more common in persons with cirrhosis (enlarged blood vessels in the oesophagus and stomach).

Another possible side effect of nonalcoholic fatty liver disease is liver cancer. According to studies, those who have nonalcoholic fatty liver disease (NAFLD) are more likely than those who do not to get liver cancer. Hepatocellular carcinoma, another name for liver cancer, develops when aberrant cells in the liver start to proliferate and divide uncontrollably.

It is unclear how exactly nonalcoholic fatty liver disease (NAFLD) raises the risk of liver cancer. On the other hand, it's thought that NAFLD-related chronic inflammation and liver damage have a role in the development of liver cancer. Furthermore, the risk of liver cancer is increased by the development of cirrhosis, which can arise from non-alcoholic fatty liver disease (NAFLD).

Early on in its development, liver cancer frequently exhibits no symptoms, making detection challenging. However, symptoms including weight loss, jaundice, and stomach pain may appear as the malignancy gets worse. Treatment methods include surgery, liver transplantation, and chemotherapy may be beneficial if liver cancer is discovered early on. The prognosis is typically bad if the cancer has progressed outside of the liver.

Non Alcoholic Fatty Liver Disease can result in cirrhosis, liver cancer, and other consequences such type 2 diabetes and cardiovascular disease. NAFLD has been linked to a higher risk of heart disease and stroke, according to research. Insulin resistance, inflammation, and oxidative stress are only a few of the complex and multiple underlying pathways that connect NAFLD to cardiovascular disease.

Moreover, type 2 diabetes and non-alcoholic fatty liver disease (NAFLD) frequently coexist, and both disorders share risk factors like insulin resistance and obesity. Increased insulin resistance and lower glycemic control can result from the metabolic abnormalities linked to diabetes being exacerbated by the presence of NAFLD.

Modifying one's lifestyle, getting medical attention, and closely monitoring oneself are all important components of a holistic approach to managing these potential consequences of nonalcoholic fatty liver disease. I stress the value of a holistic approach to healthcare and wellbeing because I am a medical doctor as well as a health and wellness coach.

This entails offering patients individualised lifestyle adjustments like consistent exercise, a balanced diet, methods for reducing stress, and enough sleep. In order to provide my patients a thorough treatment plan, I also collaborate closely with a group of professionals from other wellness and health-related sectors.

Nutrition and diet are essential for managing nonalcoholic fatty liver disease. To create individualised meal plans for my patients that encourage weight loss, increase insulin sensitivity, and lower inflammation, I collaborate with registered dietitians. In addition to promoting better liver function, a diet high in fruits, vegetables, whole grains, lean meats, and healthy fats can stop NAFLD from progressing to more severe consequences.

Along with dietary adjustments, I help my patients manage the difficulties of having a chronic illness like NAFLD by offering counselling and psychology-related approaches. A person's mental and emotional health can be greatly impacted by chronic illnesses, so it's critical to address these facets of wellness as well.

In addition, I teach my patients about complementary and alternative self-care methods like yoga, meditation, and acupuncture that can enhance general wellbeing and liver health. These methods can support better sleep, relaxation, and stress reduction—all critical for preserving liver function.

In addition, I provide my patients with coping mechanisms and self-help methods so they may properly manage their conditions. This entails giving them the knowledge and tools they need to understand the healthcare system, stand up for themselves, and choose a course of treatment.

We can significantly lower the risk of consequences like cirrhosis and liver cancer by managing non-alcoholic fatty liver disease holistically and comprehensively. We can support and guide our patients toward achieving optimal liver health and general well-being by addressing lifestyle issues, administering medical treatment, and providing support.

Preventing Liver Damage

Before we start on the path to liver health, allow me to clarify the importance of this important organ. The liver is an important organ for many processes in the body, such as metabolism, detoxification, and the production of vital proteins. On the other hand, NAFLD causes the liver to become infiltrated with extra fat deposits, which can cause damage and inflammation. In the absence of appropriate treatment and management, this illness may worsen and lead to liver cirrhosis or non-alcoholic steatohepatitis (NASH). Therefore, protecting the liver becomes crucial to our quest for general health.

1. Lifestyle Modifications:

The most important thing that NAFLD patients can do to prevent liver damage is to make the necessary lifestyle changes. These adjustments include eating a balanced diet, exercising frequently, controlling stress, and keeping a healthy weight. In order to successfully guide you, allow me to go into each of these areas:

a. Healthy Diet:

The cornerstone of your eating plan should be a diet abundant in fresh fruits, vegetables, whole grains, lean proteins, and healthy fats. For people with NAFLD, avoiding refined carbs, sugary meals, and trans and saturated fats is essential. Make a point of including foods that promote liver health, such as cruciferous vegetables, walnuts, green tea, and fatty fish (like salmon and mackerel) (such as broccoli and Brussels sprouts). Furthermore, drinking less alcohol and using water or herbal teas instead of alcohol might have a substantial positive impact on your liver.

b. Regular Physical Activity:

Exercise is crucial for maintaining a healthy weight as well as for the health of the liver. Regular exercise lowers inflammation and increases insulin sensitivity, two factors that are critical for controlling NAFLD. To maintain muscle mass and general fitness, try to get in at least 150 minutes of moderate-intensity aerobic exercise per week in addition to strength training activities. Make time for the things you enjoy doing, like dance, yoga, swimming, or brisk walking, and include them into your daily schedule.

c. Stress Management:

Stress has a significant effect on our liver as well as our general health. Chronic stress can increase the symptoms of non-alcoholic fatty liver disease (NAFLD) by releasing hormones that encourage the liver to store fat. You can effectively control your stress levels by incorporating stress-reduction practises, such as deep breathing exercises, yoga, meditation, or hobbies and activities that you enjoy. Make self-care a priority and schedule downtime for rest and renewal.

d. Maintaining a Healthy Weight:

One of the most important aspects of managing NAFLD is keeping a healthy weight. Obesity, especially fat around the abdomen, is closely linked to the onset and course of this illness. Achieving and preserving a healthy body mass index (BMI) within the range advised for your age and gender should be your major priority. A balanced diet, consistent exercise, and lifestyle changes will help you lose weight and lessen the stress on your liver.

2. Food and Diet Planning:

Food and diet planning cater to the unique requirements of NAFLD patients, whereas lifestyle adjustments cover the wider facets of a healthy lifestyle. We can provide the liver the nourishment and balance it needs to perform at its best by eating a nutritious, well-balanced diet. The following useful advice can be included into your everyday routine:

a. Portion Control:

In order to avoid consuming too many calories and to maintain a healthy weight, portion control is crucial. To make it appear as though your plate is fuller, use smaller bowls and plates. Utilize mindful eating strategies and pay attention to your body's signals of hunger and fullness. Aim for meals that are well-balanced and comprise a mix of healthy fats, carbohydrates, and protein.

b. Balanced Macronutrients:

Maintaining a balanced intake of macronutrients—carbohydrates, proteins, and fats—is essential for NAFLD patients. Pay attention to complex carbs, which offer fibre and long-lasting energy. Examples of these include whole grains and legumes. To maintain liver health, include lean proteins (fish, poultry, beans, and tofu) and healthy fats (avocado, olive oil, nuts, and seeds). Steer clear of processed carbs, saturated fats, and trans fats in excess as these might aggravate liver inflammation and damage.

c. Regular Meal Timings:

Appropriate meal time is important for controlling blood sugar and avoiding insulin spikes. Aim for two nutritious snacks and three well-balanced meals spread out throughout the day at regular intervals. Avoid going without food for extended periods of time since this might cause energy imbalances and exacerbate the symptoms of non-alcoholic fatty liver disease.

d. Hydration:

Maintaining adequate hydration promotes liver function and is vital for general health. Develop the daily practise of consuming a sufficient amount of water. This promotes easier digestion as well as the body's ability to expel impurities. You may add variety and extra health advantages by including herbal teas and infusions.

3. Counseling and Psychology-related Techniques:

When it comes to achieving liver health, the psychological health of those with nonalcoholic fatty liver disease is very important. Problems with body image, tension, and worry are frequently brought on by the difficulties in controlling this illness. I support treating these psychological factors as a health and wellness coach in order to guarantee a comprehensive strategy for managing non-alcoholic fatty liver disease. To enhance your mental health, take into account the following strategies:

a. Counseling:

Getting help from a skilled counsellor can help with stress, anxiety, and other emotional issues related to non-alcoholic fasting liver disease. A qualified counsellor can offer a secure environment where people can voice their worries, pick up coping mechanisms, and strengthen their resilience.

b. Group Support:

Connecting with others going through similar struggles might be facilitated for people with NAFLD by joining a support group or taking part in group therapy sessions. Managing the emotional components of this condition can be greatly aided by gaining support from peers, sharing experiences, and exchanging knowledge.

c. Cognitive-Behavioral Techniques:

Cognitive-behavioral methods can assist people in changing their perspective, refuting unfavourable ideas, and creating constructive coping mechanisms. Improved emotional well-being can be attained through relaxation techniques, positive self-talk, and the identification and reframing of limiting beliefs.

d. Mindfulness and Meditation:

People with NAFLD may address any excessive emotions they may be experiencing and develop a sense of awareness by engaging in mindfulness and meditation practises. Practicing mindfulness techniques (like yoga or tai chi), meditation, and deep breathing exercises can promote serenity and enhance mental health in general.

4. Self-care Alternatives and Complementary Techniques:

Examining complementary and alternative forms of self-care can provide people more tools to manage their non-alcoholic fatty liver disease (NAFLD) in addition to traditional treatments and lifestyle changes. Let's look at some choices that are worth thinking about:

a. Herbal Supplements:

A number of herbal supplements, including turmeric, dandelion, and milk thistle, have demonstrated promise in promoting liver function. Before adding any herbal supplements to your regimen, you should speak with a healthcare provider because some may interact with your current prescriptions or be contraindicated.

b. Acupuncture:

Thin needles are inserted into the body at predetermined locations during the traditional Chinese medical procedure known as acupuncture. Acupuncture therapies have been reported by some NAFLD patients to enhance liver function and relieve symptoms. More investigation is need to determine its efficacy in managing NAFLD, though.

c. Massage Therapy:

When administered by a qualified expert, massage therapy can promote liver health, reduce stress, and promote relaxation. Detoxification may be aided by methods like lymphatic drainage massage, which increase lymph flow and circulation.

d. Yoga and Tai Chi:

Practices like yoga and tai chi, with their gentle movements and emphasis on breathing, can help promote general well-being and reduce stress. In order to promote both physical and emotional well-being, think about include these mind-body workouts in your regimen.

5. Coping Strategies and Self-help Techniques:

NAFLD can be difficult to live with, but people can improve their capacity to manage it well by learning appropriate coping mechanisms and self-care practises. Here are some important pointers to remember:

a. Education and Knowledge:

Since information is power, becoming knowledgeable about NAFLD can enable you to make wise decisions about your health. To have a better understanding of your disease and treatment options, keep up with the latest research, participate in support groups, and have open communication with your healthcare provider.

b. Goal Setting and Tracking:

Having a sense of accomplishment and drive can come from setting reasonable goals and monitoring your progress. Whether your objective is to follow a suggested diet plan, increase physical activity, or lose weight, break it down into smaller, more manageable tasks to keep yourself motivated along the way.

c. Journaling:

Maintaining a journal can be an effective way to document symptoms, think back on yourself, and spot trends. Writing in a diary can help you become more self-aware and can offer insightful information for conversations with your healthcare team. You can record your food consumption, feelings, or reactions to specific therapies.

d. Building a Support System:

Having a solid support network of loved ones, friends, and medical experts is crucial for managing nonalcoholic fatty liver disease. Seek guidance from medical professionals, rely on your loved ones for support, and think about joining online communities or support groups to meet people going through similar experiences.

Never forget that every step matters when you set out to preserve liver health and stop additional harm. You get closer to optimal well-being with each lifestyle, nutritional, and self-help technique adjustment. I urge you to take hold of these useful hints and techniques and tenaciously apply them to your everyday activities. You will live the full and vibrant life you deserve as we work together to conquer non-alcoholic fatty liver disease.

The Role of Nutrition in Liver Health

NAFLD is a disorder where too much fat builds up in the liver, frequently as a result of bad dietary and lifestyle decisions. It is impacting millions of individuals globally and is getting more frequent. The good news is that with making dietary and lifestyle adjustments, NAFLD may frequently be controlled and even completely cured.

Nutrition is important for controlling nonalcoholic fatty liver disease. Our liver's condition is directly impacted by the things we eat. While some nutrients can improve liver function, others may make the situation worse. To aid in the management of nonalcoholic fatty liver disease (NAFLD), it is critical to comprehend how nutrition affects liver function and make wise dietary decisions.

A major dietary guideline for NAFLD management is to emphasise complete, unprocessed foods. This entails staying away from processed meals, which are frequently heavy in bad fats and added sugars, such as sugary drinks, fast food, and packaged snacks. These meals have the potential to exacerbate NAFLD symptoms by causing the liver to accumulate fat.

Rather, I advise my patients to consume a diet high in whole grains, fruits, vegetables, and lean meats. These meals are rich in nutrients and give the body vital minerals, vitamins, and antioxidants. They can assist liver function, lessen inflammation, and advance general wellbeing.

Specifically, I advise my patients to incorporate high-fiber foods into their diets. Fiber supports a healthy digestive system and aids in blood sugar regulation. Additionally, it lessens the amount of fat and cholesterol absorbed, which lessens the load on the liver. Fruits, vegetables, legumes, and whole grains are among the foods high in dietary fibre.

Macronutrient balance is a critical component of diet for managing non-alcoholic fatty liver disease (NAFLD). Overconsumption of carbohydrates, particularly refined carbohydrates, can lead to the buildup of fat in the liver. Rather, I suggest a well-balanced diet with lean proteins, healthy fats, and modest amounts of carbohydrates.

I advise my patients to pick complex carbohydrates over simple carbohydrates when it comes to carbohydrates. Because complex carbs digest more slowly, they contribute to stable blood sugar levels and a consistent release of energy. They are present in foods including sweet potatoes, quinoa, brown rice, and whole grains.

In order to manage NAFLD, a balanced diet must include healthy fats as well. They promote overall liver health and aid in the regulation of inflammation. Avocados, almonds, seeds, and fatty fish like mackerel and salmon are good sources of good fats.

Another essential ingredient for the health of the liver is protein. It is necessary for the regeneration and repair of liver cells. Lean protein sources like chicken, turkey, fish, tofu, and lentils are things I advise my patients to eat. Note that consuming too much protein might strain the liver, thus limits should be placed on this.

It's critical to address lifestyle issues that can affect liver function in addition to dietary modifications. Because it lowers liver fat accumulation and increases insulin sensitivity, regular exercise is essential for controlling nonalcoholic fatty liver disease (NAFLD). I advise my patients to exercise for at least 150 minutes a week at a moderate to high effort, such as cycling, swimming, or brisk walking.

Another crucial component of managing NAFLD is stress management. Liver damage and inflammation can both be exacerbated by stress. I advise my patients to make regular use of stress-reduction practises including deep breathing exercises, yoga, meditation, and mindfulness. These methods can boost general liver health, lower stress levels, and encourage relaxation.

In summary, it is impossible to overestimate the importance of diet for liver health. Dietary adjustments are essential for controlling non-alcoholic fatty liver disease and supporting liver health in those who have it. Individuals can promote liver function and minimise inflammation by focusing on complete, unprocessed foods, such as fruits, vegetables, whole grains, lean meats, and healthy fats. The management of NAFLD might also be enhanced by adding frequent exercise and stress-reduction strategies. People can improve their general well-being and take charge of their liver health by adopting a holistic approach to healthcare and wellbeing.

Exercise and Lifestyle Modifications

There is no quick fix or miracle medication for treating Non Alcoholic Fatty Liver Disease (NAFLD). It necessitates an all-encompassing strategy that targets the disease's underlying causes and fosters long-term healthiness. Lifestyle changes and frequent exercise are two of this approach's main tenets.

It has long been known that exercise is an effective way to preserve and enhance general health. In the case of NAFLD, it is the same. Regular exercise has been demonstrated to help lower liver fat, enhance liver function, and stop the disease's progression.

Exercise helps people with non-alcoholic fatty liver disease (NAFLD) in multiple ways. First off, one prevalent underlying problem in NAFLD is insulin resistance, which can be reduced with physical activity. The term "insulin resistance" describes the body's diminished capacity to react to the insulin hormone, which controls blood sugar levels. Blood insulin levels rise when insulin resistance occurs because the body's cells become less responsive to the actions of insulin. This may be one factor in the liver's fat buildup.

Frequent exercise increases insulin sensitivity, which facilitates the body's more effective use of insulin. This lessens the buildup of fat in the liver and also aids in blood sugar regulation. Moreover, exercise promotes the body's breakdown of fat reserves, including the liver, which lowers the amount of fat in the liver.

Exercise directly improves liver health in addition to its effects on fat metabolism and insulin sensitivity. It has been shown that physical activity lowers hepatic inflammation, which is a major factor in the advancement of NAFLD. Additionally, it encourages the synthesis of antioxidants, which shield liver cells from oxidative damage. Exercise has also been demonstrated to raise liver enzyme levels, which suggests better liver function.

How much exercise is sufficient, then? For those with non-alcoholic fatty liver disease (NAFLD), the American Association for the Study of Liver Diseases suggests 150 minutes or 75 minutes of moderate-intensity aerobic activity each week. This can be accomplished by engaging in any type of aerobic exercise that raises your heart rate, such as jogging, cycling, swimming, or fast walking. To enhance total body composition and muscle strength, the regimen should include strength training exercises at least twice a week.

Exercise is an essential part of addressing non-alcoholic fatty liver disease (NAFLD), but for best effects, it should be paired with other lifestyle changes. Eating a healthy, balanced diet is one of the most important lifestyle adjustments that should be made. Lean protein, whole grains, fruits, vegetables, and healthy fats can all contribute to a diet that lowers liver fat and enhances liver function in general.

Refined carbohydrates, bad fats, and added sweets should all be consumed in moderation as they can also lead to the buildup of liver fat. Since alcohol can exacerbate liver impairment, it should be absolutely avoided. Including some foods and supplements that have been demonstrated to help NAFLD may also be helpful; examples include coffee, green tea, fish oil, and a few herbs and spices.

Moreover, getting enough sleep and managing stress are crucial components of managing NAFLD. Finding good coping mechanisms for stress and making sure you get enough sleep and recuperation are important because chronic stress and sleep deprivation can accelerate the disease's course.

I collaborate closely with my patients as a physician and health and wellness coach to help them put these lifestyle changes into practise and develop a thorough strategy for managing their non-alcoholic fatty liver disease (NAFLD). I am aware that implementing these adjustments can be difficult, particularly in the face of a chronic illness like NAFLD. For this reason, I assemble a team of professionals from several health and wellness domains, such as dietitians, psychologists, and practitioners of alternative medicine, for my patients. We work together to offer my patients the resources and assistance they require to make long-lasting lifestyle changes.

It's critical to treat any underlying medical issues that might be influencing the onset or progression of NAFLD in addition to exercise and lifestyle changes. With the assistance of medical professionals, conditions including obesity, diabetes, high blood pressure, and high cholesterol should be appropriately addressed. Prescription drugs may be used to treat these ailments and lower the chance of more liver damage.

In summary, lifestyle changes and consistent exercise are essential for the management of nonalcoholic fatty liver disease. Exercise enhances liver function, lowers liver fat level, and increases insulin sensitivity. To maximise liver health, lifestyle changes including stress reduction, a balanced diet, and enough sleep are crucial. You may take charge of your NAFLD and enhance your general health and well-being by implementing these adjustments into your everyday routine. Never forget that you can start living a better life and making positive changes at any time. Your liver will be appreciative.

Chapter 3: Understanding Non Alcoholic Fatty Liver Disease

Non Alcoholic Fatty Liver Disease: The Silent Epidemic

Throughout history, Alcoholic Liver Disease—the alcoholic analogue of NAFLD—has frequently eclipsed it (ALD). However, NAFLD has become a secret epidemic that affects people of all ages, genders, and races due to shifting food habits, lifestyle changes, and the growing global epidemic of obesity and metabolic syndrome. Simple steatosis, or the buildup of fat in the liver, to nonalcoholic steatohepatitis (NASH), which is marked by inflammation and destruction to the liver cells, are all included in this category of chronic liver disease.

The past few decades have seen a sharp increase in the prevalence of NAFLD, which is consistent with the global rise in obesity rates. A quarter of the world's population is thought to be affected by NAFLD, which has an unparalleled prevalence, according to several studies. As much as 35–40 percent of people may be affected in various areas, including the Middle East, South America, and Asia.

Since type 2 diabetes, obesity, dyslipidemia, hypertension, and other metabolic disorders are closely linked to non-alcoholic fatty liver disease (NAFLD), the ramifications of this silent epidemic are extensive. NAFLD is a complex condition that necessitates all-encompassing care because these comorbidities frequently group together and contribute to the disease's progression.

Being asymptomatic in the early stages, when people might not realise they have NAFLD until problems start to occur, is one of the biggest obstacles to treating the condition. Unfortunately, NAFLD is frequently disregarded in standard medical evaluations, with many physicians being unable to identify the symptoms and indicators. Screening and detection are therefore crucial.

It has been demonstrated by recent study that children and adolescents are increasingly being affected by non-alcoholic fatty liver disease (NAFLD). This worrying trend is mostly due to the growth in childhood obesity rates. These people's future health is affected by the early onset of the illness because NAFLD has been found to be a substantial risk factor for the development of cirrhosis, severe liver disease, and even hepatocellular cancer.

In addition, NAFLD places a massive financial strain on both patients and healthcare systems. Effective prevention and management techniques are desperately needed, as evidenced by the high expenses of detecting, treating, and managing NAFLD as well as the possible long-term consequences and decreased quality of life.

Researchers and medical experts are investigating the pathogenesis of non-alcoholic fatty liver disease (NAFLD) and possible treatment strategies in light of the disease's widespread effect. Developing focused treatment plans and preventative actions requires an understanding of the mechanisms causing nonalcoholic fatty liver disease (NAFLD).

There is a clear correlation between insulin resistance and non-alcoholic fatty liver disease (NAFLD), and correcting insulin resistance through dietary changes and physical activity can greatly enhance liver health. Moreover, research has demonstrated that reducing weight with a mix of exercise and dietary modifications can enhance liver function and lower liver fat.

All the same, it's crucial to remember that treating NAFLD calls for a comprehensive strategy. A healthy lifestyle, which includes eating well, exercising, reducing stress, and getting enough sleep, is essential for both preventing and treating NAFLD. To further improve overall results, comorbidities including diabetes and dyslipidemia must be addressed.

In my capacity as a physician and health and wellness coach, my colleagues and I work hard to offer complete care and support to people with non-alcoholic fatty liver disease (NAFLD). We are aware of the particular difficulties every patient has, and we make every effort to create individualised management programmes that cater to their individual requirements.

In conclusion, non-alcoholic fatty liver disease is becoming increasingly common and has significant effects on people's lives as well as global healthcare systems. This invisible epidemic needs to be addressed immediately and requires a thorough strategy to care and prevention. We can fight the silent pandemic of nonalcoholic fatty liver disease (NAFLD) and enhance the health and well-being of those who are impacted by this chronic liver disease by implementing lifestyle changes, early identification, and focused therapies.

The Two Types of Non Alcoholic Fatty Liver Disease

The milder kind of NAFLD is called non-alcoholic fatty liver disease (NAFL). It is distinguished by hepatic fat accumulation without appreciable liver cell injury or inflammation. NAFL usually does not create apparent symptoms, hence it is frequently misdiagnosed. That does not, however, imply that it should be ignored. Research has indicated that in certain people, NAFL can develop into NASH, a more severe form of NAFLD.

NASH, or non-alcoholic steatohepatitis, is the more severe type of NAFLD. In addition to fat buildup in the liver, it is characterised by inflammation and damage to the liver cells. In contrast to NAFL, NASH can result in symptoms including jaundice, exhaustion, and stomach pain that are apparent. In addition, it may result in side effects like cirrhosis, liver fibrosis, or even liver cancer. Early NASH diagnosis and treatment are therefore essential to halting more liver damage and its related consequences.

Although the precise mechanisms behind the development of NASH and NAFL are still unclear, a number of factors have been suggested as possible causes. These include excessive blood triglyceride and cholesterol levels, obesity, insulin resistance, and persistent inflammation. Type 2 diabetes and metabolic syndrome, in particular, as well as genetic factors, can raise the chance of developing NAFLD, especially NASH.

It can be difficult to diagnose NAFLD and tell the difference between NAFL and NASH. It is frequently required to perform a thorough medical history, physical examination, and laboratory tests, such as imaging investigations and liver function tests. To determine the extent of inflammation and liver damage, liver biopsies can also be carried out; however, as they are invasive, they are typically saved for situations in which the diagnosis is still unclear.

Making changes to one's lifestyle and taking care of underlying risk factors are key components of NAFLD treatment. For both NAFL and NASH, weight loss achieved through a mix of dietary modifications and consistent exercise is the cornerstone of treatment. It is advised to consume less alcohol, added sweets, saturated fats, and whole grains while increasing fruits, vegetables, and lean proteins in your diet. A referral to a licenced dietitian may be helpful in some circumstances in order to create a customised food plan and offer continuing assistance.

Exercise is essential for promoting liver health in general and weight loss in particular. Frequent exercise lowers blood cholesterol levels, decreases inflammation, increases insulin sensitivity, and helps people lose weight. It is advised to use resistance training to increase muscle strength in addition to 150 minutes or more of moderate-intensity aerobic activity each week.

To treat particular elements of non-alcoholic fatty liver disease (NAFLD), doctors may also prescribe certain drugs. These include lipid-lowering therapies that lower cholesterol and triglyceride levels and insulin sensitizers that improve glucose control. To ascertain the long-term safety and effectiveness of these drugs, more study is necessary in this area of NAFLD medication use.

It's crucial to remember that treating NAFLD calls for a multidisciplinary strategy. In my capacity as a physician and health and wellness coach, my colleagues and I collaborate closely with patients to develop a thorough treatment strategy. Along with advice on diet and exercise, this also includes counselling, psychology-related techniques to support behavioural changes, self-care strategies, self-help techniques, and coping mechanisms to address the emotional and psychological aspects of managing non-alcoholic fatty liver disease (NAFLD).

To sum up, non-alcoholic fatty liver disease (NAFLD) is a common illness that includes non-alcoholic steatohepatitis and non-alcoholic fatty liver (NAFL) (NASH). The milder type, known as NAFL, is characterised by hepatic fat buildup without a large amount of inflammation or damage to the liver cells. On the other hand, NASH is more aggressive, causing fat accumulation along with inflammation and damage to liver cells. It is imperative to identify and treat NASH early in order to stop more liver damage and its related consequences. The mainstay of treatment is changing one's lifestyle, which includes eating differently, exercising frequently, and losing weight. To effectively manage nonalcoholic fatty liver disease (NAFLD) and improve overall liver function, a multidisciplinary approach including medical specialists and experts in health and wellness is essential.

Causes and Risk Factors

The onset of NAFLD is mostly influenced by genetics. Studies have indicated that fatty liver disease risk may be elevated by specific gene variations. Insulin signalling, lipid metabolism, and inflammation are all regulated by these genes. Changes in these genes may result in an inability to adequately metabolise and store fat, which may cause the liver to become too obese. The development and severity of NAFLD can still be influenced by other factors and lifestyle decisions, even while genetics may predispose a person to the condition.

The onset of NAFLD is also significantly influenced by lifestyle decisions. Consuming a diet high in calories, especially one heavy in refined carbs and saturated fats, can cause the liver to become obese. This is because these foods cause an excess of calories to be turned into triglycerides, which are subsequently deposited in the liver. Overindulging in calories on a regular basis can cause the liver's capacity to break down and eliminate these triglycerides, which can lead to the development of fatty liver disease.

NAFLD can also develop as a result of sedentary lifestyles and low levels of physical activity. Frequent exercise has been demonstrated to enhance hepatic fat metabolism and insulin sensitivity. On the other hand, a sedentary lifestyle can result in insulin resistance and a decreased liver's capacity to process and eliminate fat. This may have an impact on the onset and course of NAFLD.

NAFLD development is significantly influenced by underlying medical disorders as well. Fatty liver disease is strongly linked to the emergence of conditions like obesity, type 2 diabetes, and metabolic syndrome. Insulin resistance, which affects the liver's capacity to control the synthesis and storage of lipids, is frequently associated with several disorders. Furthermore, the development of NAFLD and liver damage can be further exacerbated by chronic inflammation, which is frequently observed in these circumstances.

Recalling that NAFLD is a complex disease—that is, one in which several factors frequently combine to contribute to its development—is crucial. People who possess specific genetic variants can be more vulnerable to the negative consequences of leading a sedentary or unhealthy lifestyle. Likewise, the influence of lifestyle decisions on the liver might be intensified by preexisting medical disorders. Consequently, all of these contributory factors should be addressed in a comprehensive approach to controlling NAFLD.

I extensively collaborate with patients in my practise to pinpoint the precise causes of their non-alcoholic fatty liver disease (NAFLD). This frequently entails taking a complete medical history, determining their genetic susceptibility, analysing their food and exercise habits, and doing an underlying health problem screening. We are able to create individualised treatment programmes that cater to the particular needs of every patient by adopting a holistic approach.

One of the mainstays of managing NAFLD is changing one's lifestyle. In close collaboration with my patients, I create individualised food and exercise regimens that support liver function and lessen fat storage. Reducing calorie intake, emphasising complete, unprocessed foods, consuming more fruits and vegetables, and avoiding refined carbs and saturated fats are some ways to do this. To increase insulin sensitivity and enhance the liver's breakdown of fat, regular physical activity is also advised, including aerobic and muscular training.

In addition to modifying one's lifestyle, treating underlying medical issues is essential for managing non-alcoholic fatty liver disease (NAFLD). Losing weight is frequently an important part of treatment for people with obesity or metabolic syndrome. Combining a healthy diet, regular exercise, and sometimes medication can help achieve this. Similarly, it's critical for people with type 2 diabetes to control their blood sugar levels through medication and lifestyle modifications. We can lessen the effects of these underlying medical issues on the liver and enhance liver health in general by taking care of them.

In summary, a mix of genetics, lifestyle decisions, and underlying medical issues contribute to the development of non-alcoholic fatty liver disease. It is crucial to comprehend these elements in order to create efficient management plans for this complicated illness. We may work toward enhancing liver function and eventually reaching full NAFLD control by adopting a comprehensive strategy that includes nutrition, exercise, and the treatment of underlying medical issues.

Metabolic Syndrome and Non Alcoholic Fatty Liver Disease

Being a physician and a health and wellness coach, I am always reminded of how vital lifestyle decisions and general health are to our entire wellbeing. Non Alcoholic Fatty Liver Disease (NAFLD) is one ailment that has become more common in recent years. It is closely associated with a condition called metabolic syndrome. We will examine the relationship between metabolic syndrome and non-alcoholic fatty liver disease (NAFLD) in this chapter, as well as the reciprocal effects of these two disorders.

We must first identify and examine each condition separately in order to fully comprehend the connection between metabolic syndrome and non-alcoholic fatty liver disease. A group of related disorders known as metabolic syndrome raise the risk of diabetes, stroke, and cardiovascular disease. These ailments include low levels of HDL (good) cholesterol, high blood pressure, high blood sugar, high triglyceride levels, and abdominal obesity. Fatal weight gain, sedentary lifestyles, and poor diets are common causes of metabolic syndrome.

However, NAFLD is a disease that is not brought on by excessive alcohol consumption; rather, it is characterised by the buildup of fat in the liver. It is regarded as a chronic illness and the primary global cause of liver-related morbidity and mortality. NAFLD is frequently linked to sedentary behaviour, obesity, insulin resistance, and metabolic syndrome.

The underlying risk factors that both metabolic syndrome and non-alcoholic fatty liver disease share are what link them. For example, obesity is a major factor in the development of both illnesses. Excess body fat, especially visceral fat that builds up around the abdominal organs, is linked to chronic inflammation, dyslipidemia, and insulin resistance—all of which are major risk factors for metabolic syndrome and non-alcoholic fatty liver disease (NAFLD).

One further similarity that exists between NAFLD and metabolic syndrome is insulin resistance. Excess body fat causes the body's cells to become less sensitive to insulin, which raises blood sugar levels and increases the risk of type 2 diabetes. Additionally, hepatic lipogenesis—the process by which the liver makes fat—is encouraged by insulin resistance. The onset and advancement of NAFLD are further aided by this increased fat production.

Moreover, dyslipidemia, a disorder marked by elevated lipid levels, is common in NAFLD and metabolic syndrome. Individuals with dyslipidemia frequently have high triglyceride and low HDL cholesterol levels, which are indicative of the disorder. Atherosclerosis, a disorder characterised by the buildup of fatty deposits in the arteries, is facilitated by the aberrant lipid profiles found in metabolic syndrome and non-alcoholic fatty liver disease (NAFLD), which raises the risk of heart disease.

NAFLD and metabolic syndrome are also related to chronic inflammation. The body's natural reaction to damage or infection is inflammation. On the other hand, persistent inflammation has been linked to the onset and advancement of several illnesses, such as metabolic syndrome and nonalcoholic fatty liver disease (NAFLD). Obesity and metabolic syndrome patients have more adipose tissue, which can release pro-inflammatory molecules called adipokines. These molecules can exacerbate liver fibrosis and inflammation, ultimately resulting in cirrhosis and liver failure.

Although it is evident that metabolic syndrome and non-alcoholic fatty liver disease (NAFLD) have similar risk factors and a close interaction, it is equally important to recognise that their influence is reciprocal. Because the underlying insulin resistance and dyslipidemia associated with metabolic syndrome foster an environment that is conducive to hepatic fat storage, metabolic syndrome can predispose people to developing non-alcoholic fatty liver disease (NAFLD). Alternatively, the existence of non-alcoholic fatty liver disease (NAFLD) might exacerbate metabolic syndrome by sustaining insulin resistance and dyslipidemia, hence exacerbating the progression of cardiovascular illness and type 2 diabetes.

Apart from their direct connections, metabolic syndrome and non-alcoholic fasting diabetes mellitus are linked to several other health issues that intensify their combined effects. Among these problems are chronic renal disease, hypertension, type 2 diabetes, and cardiovascular disease. Thus, treating and controlling metabolic syndrome and nonalcoholic fatty liver disease (NAFLD) is essential not only for liver health but also for general health and disease prevention.

In my capacity as a health and wellness coach, I stress the significance of treating these diseases holistically. Making changes to one's lifestyle is essential for managing and preventing metabolic syndrome and NAFLD. This include consuming a healthy, balanced diet, exercising frequently, controlling stress, getting enough sleep, giving up smoking, and abstaining from excessive alcohol use. These alterations in lifestyle can help decrease the buildup of liver fat, lower cholesterol, decrease belly fat, and increase insulin sensitivity.

Comprehensive management necessitates the integration of diverse health and wellness specialists' knowledge. This entails collaborating with registered dietitians to create customised meal programmes that satisfy dietary needs and treat particular ailments. Furthermore, treatments like cognitive-behavioral therapy and stress reduction methods can be helpful in removing obstacles to leading a healthy lifestyle.

Effective management of metabolic syndrome and nonalcoholic fatty liver disease (NAFLD) requires an understanding of their complex interaction. Through the identification and management of common risk factors, a comprehensive strategy, and expert coaching, people may take charge of their health, halt the advancement of these disorders, and enhance their overall quality of life.

We will examine how food affects metabolic syndrome and nonalcoholic fatty liver disease (NAFLD) in the upcoming chapter, with particular attention to dietary suggestions that can reverse insulin resistance and support liver health. Never forget that information is power. With the correct knowledge and resources, you may become an expert in managing NAFLD and metabolic syndrome.

Understanding Insulin Resistance

It's critical to understand the physiological function of insulin in our bodies in order to fully appreciate the implications of insulin resistance in non-alcoholic fatty liver disease. When blood sugar levels rise, the pancreas releases the hormone insulin. Its principal job is to make glucose easier for cells to absorb and use, so the body can keep blood sugar levels steady.

In a healthy person, insulin binds to insulin receptors on the surface of the cell, starting a series of events that let glucose enter the cell and either be used immediately as energy or stored as glycogen for later use. On the other hand, when a person has insulin resistance, their cell receptors lose their sensitivity to insulin's signals. Insulin levels in the blood rise as a result of the body trying to compensate for this resistance by producing more insulin.

Insulin controls blood sugar levels and is essential for lipid metabolism, which is why there is a link between insulin resistance and non-alcoholic fatty liver disease (NAFLD). The body's capacity to appropriately control fat metabolism is hampered when insulin resistance sets up. Triglycerides build up and non-alcoholic fatty liver disease (NAFLD) develops as a result of increased fat storage in the liver.

Several facets of liver function are significantly impacted by insulin resistance as well. Inflammatory cytokines and free fatty acids are produced more readily by it, and this can cause damage and inflammation to the liver. In addition, it throws off the equilibrium between the breakdown and synthesis of liver fat, which eventually encourages the growth of liver fibrosis and the advancement of nonalcoholic steatohepatitis (NASH) and cirrhosis, two more severe stages of NAFLD.

In order to treat NAFLD completely, managing insulin resistance is essential. Fortunately, people can modify their lifestyle in a number of ways to increase their sensitivity to insulin and lessen the damaging effects of insulin resistance on their liver.

Adopting a nutritious diet is crucial, first and foremost. Blood sugar levels can be stabilised, inflammation can be decreased, and liver function can be improved with a diet high in whole, unprocessed foods including fruits, vegetables, lean proteins, and healthy fats. Refined carbs, sugary drinks, and trans fats should be consumed in moderation since they can worsen insulin resistance and hinder the development of non-alcoholic fatty liver disease (NAFLD).

Another important factor in controlling insulin resistance is regular physical activity. By increasing muscle glucose absorption and decreasing the buildup of liver fat, exercise helps increase insulin sensitivity. It can be very helpful to manage insulin resistance and lower the risk of NAFLD progression by partaking in exercises like high-intensity interval training, strength training, and aerobic activity.

Weight control is a crucial component of managing insulin resistance in addition to dietary and exercise therapies. Insulin resistance and non-alcoholic fatty liver disease are closely linked to excess body weight, especially abdominal fat. Consequently, insulin sensitivity and liver function can be greatly enhanced by reaching and maintaining a healthy body weight by a mix of dietary adjustments, physical activity, and behaviour modification strategies.

To address insulin resistance, certain medicines may also be administered. For instance, metformin is frequently prescribed to people with type 2 diabetes and prediabetes in order to enhance insulin sensitivity and glycemic management. Certain situations may also warrant the consideration of other drugs, such as thiazolidinediones; however, due to potential side effects, their use should be closely monitored.

Finally, in order to properly manage this increasingly common condition, it is imperative to comprehend the role that insulin resistance plays in the onset and progression of non-alcoholic fatty liver

disease. Insulin resistance affects lipid metabolism as well as glucose metabolism, which causes a build-up of fat in the liver and eventual damage to the liver. People can increase their insulin sensitivity and lessen the negative effects of insulin resistance on their liver health by implementing a comprehensive strategy that includes weight control, regular exercise, healthy lifestyle changes, and possibly pharmacological therapy. To create a customised management strategy that tackles every facet of non-alcoholic fatty liver disease (NAFLD) and insulin resistance, close collaboration with healthcare experts—such as nutritionists, health coaches, and primary care physicians—is essential. When we work together, we can eliminate the burden of non-alcoholic fatty liver disease in the future.

Inflammation and Oxidative Stress

Nonalcoholic Fatty Liver Disease is characterised by the onset and advancement of inflammation and oxidative damage (NAFLD). Effective management and treatment of the illness depend on an understanding of the effects of these processes. This chapter will examine the complex relationship that exists between oxidative stress, inflammation, and non-alcoholic fatty liver disease (NAFLD) and will also discuss ways to mitigate these effects for improved liver health.

Detoxification and lipid metabolism are just two of the many metabolic processes carried out by the liver, an essential organ. When too much fat accumulates in the liver, as it does in people with non-alcoholic fatty liver disease (NAFLD), inflammation and oxidative stress result.

The body's normal reaction to damage or infection is inflammation. To restore damaged tissues, certain chemicals and immune cells are released. On the other hand, persistent inflammation may have a deleterious impact on the liver and accelerate the development of NAFLD. Studies reveal elevated levels of inflammatory markers, including tumour necrosis factor-alpha (TNF-α) and C-reactive protein (CRP), in people with non-alcoholic fatty liver disease (NAFLD) (TNF-alpha).

Conversely, oxidative stress results from an imbalance between the body's antioxidant defences and the generation of reactive oxygen species (ROS). Although the body produces ROS naturally throughout many metabolic activities, diseases like NAFLD can cause an overabundance of these molecules. These too many ROS can cause inflammation and harm to liver cells.

In NAFLD, oxidative stress and inflammation frequently coexist and feed one another into a vicious cycle. Increased ROS production following inflammation fuels more inflammation. The damage to liver cells is sustained by this cycle, which also makes NAFLD worse.

It takes a multimodal strategy to lessen the effects of oxidative stress and inflammation on NAFLD. A thorough management strategy can include the following essential techniques:

1. Dietary modifications: For NAFLD to be managed, a nutritious, well-balanced diet is crucial. Consuming foods high in antioxidants, such as whole grains, fruits, and vegetables, can assist in preventing oxidative stress. Furthermore, since processed meals, sugar-filled drinks, and trans fats exacerbate inflammation and liver damage, it is imperative to stay away from them.

2. Weight management: Reducing excess weight can significantly improve liver health, as obesity is a substantial risk factor for NAFLD. In those with non-alcoholic fatty liver disease (NAFLD), gradual weight loss achieved by combining a nutritious diet with frequent exercise has been found to lower oxidative stress and inflammation.

3. Regular exercise: Regular physical activity offers immediate anti-inflammatory benefits in addition to helping with weight management. It has been demonstrated that exercise increases antioxidant capacity and lowers inflammatory marker levels in NAFLD patients.

4. Stress management: Oxidative stress and inflammation might worsen under long-term stress. The negative effects of stress on liver function can be mitigated by using stress management practises such deep breathing exercises, mindfulness meditation, and routine relaxation.

5. Nutritional supplements: Promising results have been observed in lowering oxidative stress and inflammation in NAFLD patients who use certain dietary supplements. The most researched and found to have positive benefits on liver function include omega-3 fatty acids, vitamin E, and N-acetyl cysteine (NAC).

6. Herbal remedies: For their hepatoprotective qualities, some plants have been utilised for a long time, including milk thistle and

turmeric. These herbs can lessen liver damage and improve overall liver health because of their anti-inflammatory and antioxidant qualities.

7. Medications: Medication may occasionally be recommended to treat NAFLD-related inflammation and oxidative damage. But because they could have negative effects, these should always be used under a doctor's supervision.

8. Regular monitoring: Frequent imaging examinations and liver function tests can be used to track the development of nonalcoholic fatty liver disease (NAFLD) and evaluate the success of anti-inflammatory and anti-oxidative stressive therapies.

It is crucial to remember that NAFLD care needs to be customised for each patient, taking into consideration their particular situation. To guarantee a comprehensive and individualised strategy, it is recommended to collaborate closely with healthcare experts who specialise in managing non-alcoholic fry syndrome (NAFLD).

In summary, oxidative stress and inflammation play a major role in the onset and development of NAFLD. Effective management of this disease requires an understanding of their impact and the implementation of interventions to mitigate their effects. NAFLD patients can take charge of their liver health and halt the disease's progression by changing their lifestyle, using particular supplements and herbal therapies as needed, and seeing a doctor on a regular basis.

The Gut-Liver Axis

We must examine the complex web of interactions that exist between these two essential organs in greater detail in order to comprehend the gut-liver axis. The gastrointestinal tract, sometimes referred to as the gut, is in charge of breaking down and absorbing nutrients from the food we eat. Trillions of microorganisms called the gut microbiota reside there and are essential to preserving gut health.

A varied population of bacteria, viruses, fungus, and other microorganisms make up the gut microbiota. Each of these microscopic residents has a distinct function in a variety of physiological processes, and they coexist in a delicate equilibrium. They support the synthesis of vitamins, aid in the breakdown of complex carbohydrates, control immunological response, and ward off dangerous infections. However, there can be serious repercussions for human health, especially the liver's health, if this delicate equilibrium is upset.

The liver is an important organ that keeps the body functioning in many ways. It stores vital nutrients, metabolises poisons and medicines, and detoxifies dangerous chemicals. It also creates bile to aid with digesting. Liver illnesses, such as non-alcoholic fatty liver disease, can arise when the liver is overloaded with toxins or encounters other obstacles (NAFLD).

Overabundance fat builds up in the liver as a defining feature of nonalcoholic fatty liver disease (NAFLD). It is frequently linked to metabolic syndrome, insulin resistance, and obesity. It is obvious that gut health has a major impact on the development of nonalcoholic fatty liver disease (NAFLD), even though the precise mechanisms underlying its onset are not entirely known.

Studies have indicated that dysbiosis, or imbalances in the gut microbiota, may have a role in the onset and development of non-alcoholic fatty liver disease (NAFLD). Increased gut permeability brought on by dysbiosis can make it possible for dangerous chemicals like bacterial endotoxins to enter the bloodstream. These endotoxins set off an immunological reaction that results in inflammation, which damages liver cells and accelerates the onset of liver disorders.

Moreover, bile acids are necessary for the breakdown and absorption of fats, and dysbiosis might affect their synthesis and metabolism. Changes in the metabolism of bile acids can cause an imbalance in the metabolism of lipids, which can lead to the buildup of fat in the liver.

Therefore, addressing these imbalances and improving gut health are critical to managing non-alcoholic fatty liver disease (NAFLD). I support a holistic approach to healthcare and wellness as a medical doctor and health and wellness coach. We can assist patients in achieving the best possible health outcomes by treating them with a thorough and integrated approach.

In my practise, I create individualised treatment regimens for NAFLD patients in close collaboration with my team of specialists from several health and wellness domains. Our approach's emphasis on lifestyle changes is one of its main components. We teach our patients the value of stress reduction, a balanced diet, frequent exercise, and enough sleep.

In terms of nutrition, we stress the importance of consuming a diet high in whole foods and nutrients. This consists of an abundance of entire grains, fruits, vegetables, lean meats, and healthy fats. Additionally, since processed meals, sugar-filled drinks, and trans and saturated fats might deteriorate liver health, we advise our patients to minimise their intake of these items.

Furthermore, we frequently suggest particular dietary changes that have been demonstrated to improve gut health. Foods high in probiotics and prebiotics, like kimchi, sauerkraut, kefir, and yoghurt, can aid in reestablishing the proper balance of gut flora. These meals supply the essential nutrients and good bacteria that can aid in the healing of the gut and lower inflammation.

In certain situations, we could also advise using nutritional supplements to help maintain gut health. Patients who may suffer from severe dysbiosis or who cannot eat enough foods high in probiotics may benefit from taking probiotic supplements. Furthermore, it has been demonstrated that supplements containing glutamine, aloe vera, and turmeric have anti-inflammatory properties and can aid in the repair of gut epithelial cells.

Our treatment regimens often include counselling and psychology-related techniques in addition to nutritional measures. We are aware that NAFLD has psychological and emotional effects in addition to its medical ones. Emotions like as guilt, embarrassment, and frustration are common in NAFLD patients. We assist them in navigating their path to healing and self-acceptance by giving them the essential emotional support and teaching them coping mechanisms.

Including complementary and alternative self-care approaches is just another crucial component of our treatment plan. It has been demonstrated that methods like yoga, meditation, and acupuncture have a significant impact in lowering stress and improving general wellbeing. These methods can help patients better control their stress levels, get better sleep, and feel better mentally and emotionally all around.

To sum up, maintaining optimal gut health is essential for managing non-alcoholic fatty liver disease. The numerous connections within the gut-liver axis can have a substantial impact on the health of the liver. We can help our patients achieve full control of non-alcoholic fatty liver disease (NAFLD) by comprehending this relationship and putting into practise comprehensive treatment strategies that emphasise nutritional interventions, self-care measures, counselling, and lifestyle modifications. I am dedicated to inspiring my patients and assisting them in leading better and happier lives as a healthcare professional and wellness coach.

The Role of Hormones in Non Alcoholic Fatty Liver Disease

As we begin, let's take a closer look at insulin, the hormone that drives NAFLD. Insulin is the hormone that controls blood sugar levels, as we all know, but its effects go well beyond that. The metabolism and storage of fat are significantly influenced by insulin. Our bodies convert carbs into glucose, which causes the pancreas to release insulin when we eat them. Glucose is subsequently transported into our cells by insulin and consumed as fuel. But chronically high insulin levels can cause fat to build up in the liver, as they frequently do in people with type 2 diabetes or insulin resistance.

The emergence of NAFLD is strongly correlated with insulin resistance and increased insulin levels, according to numerous research. Researchers discovered that those with NAFLD had far higher fasting insulin levels than people without the condition in one study that was published in the Journal of Hepatology. Moreover, increased liver enzyme levels and the buildup of liver fat—two characteristics common of NAFLD—were linked to these raised insulin levels.

However, NAFLD is not solely caused by insulin. Leptin is an additional hormone that merits consideration. Fat cells release the hormone leptin, which is essential for controlling hunger and energy balance. Its primary job is to interact with the brain in order to reduce hunger and boost energy expenditure. Nonetheless, a condition known as leptin resistance arises in obesity and insulin resistance conditions, which are frequently observed in people with NAFLD. In other words, even with high amounts of leptin, the body gets insensitive to its effects, which causes an insatiable hunger and overindulgence in food.

Leptin resistance has been linked in numerous studies to the onset and development of non-alcoholic fatty liver disease. Emphasizing the critical function leptin plays in liver health, researchers showed in a study published in the journal Cell Metabolism that mice lacking the leptin receptor in their liver developed severe fatty liver disease. In addition, human research indicates that NAFLD patients had greater leptin levels than healthy people, which may indicate a connection between leptin dysregulation and the onset of the illness.

Let's now discuss the hormone adiponectin, which has anti-inflammatory and insulin-sensitizing qualities. The main source and secretor of adiponectin is adipose tissue, and there is an inverse relationship between adiponectin levels and body fat percentage. According to numerous studies, people with NAFLD have far lower adiponectin levels than people without the condition. Increased oxidative stress, insulin resistance, and liver inflammation have all been linked to this drop in adiponectin levels, and these factors all aid in the onset and development of nonalcoholic fatty liver disease (NAFLD).

Higher adiponectin levels were linked to a lower risk of developing non-alcoholic fatty liver disease (NAFLD) in a large cohort of women, according to a study published in the Journal of Clinical Endocrinology and Metabolism. The results of this study imply that increasing adiponectin levels may prevent the onset of NAFLD.

Even if in recent years our understanding of the role of hormones in NAFLD has improved rapidly, there is still more to learn. On the other hand, it is evident that hormones like adiponectin, insulin, and leptin play a major role in the initiation and advancement of liver disease.

I help my patients control their non-alcoholic fatty liver disease (NAFLD) by using a comprehensive approach. I offer psychological treatments and counselling in addition to lifestyle changes like regular exercise and a balanced diet to address any underlying emotional issues that might be causing the disease to worsen. Furthermore, I think that optimising hormone levels through focused medicines and interventions is really important. With the amazing outcomes of this holistic approach, my patients are equipped with the knowledge and skills necessary to take back control of their liver health.

69

In summary, the importance of hormones in NAFLD cannot be overstated. Adiponectin, leptin, and insulin all have critical functions in the onset and development of this liver disease. We can enable people to take control of their liver health and eventually attain full non-alcoholic fatty liver disease management by comprehending the complex interactions between these hormones and putting comprehensive therapies into practise.

Chapter 4: Medical Management of Non Alcoholic Fatty Liver Disease

Diagnosis and Assessment

Chapter 4: The Diagnostic Journey

As a physician and health and wellness advisor, I have guided innumerable people through the difficult process of identifying and treating nonalcoholic fatty liver disease (NAFLD). I will walk you through the intricacies of the diagnostic process in this chapter, illuminating the different tests and techniques that may be used to precisely detect and evaluate this illness. Whether you are a worried patient looking for information or a healthcare practitioner trying to learn more, this chapter will provide you the tools you need to confidently start the diagnostic process.

4.1 A Historical Timeline: Understanding the Evolution of Diagnosis

Understanding the historical context that has influenced our understanding of non-alcoholic fatty liver disease (NAFLD) is crucial before exploring the present diagnostic methodology. This liver condition, which was formerly thought to be uncommon, has dramatically increased in frequency over the past few decades, mostly due to the global obesity and sedentary lifestyle epidemic.

Through postmortem research, NAFLD was first identified as a separate entity in the 1970s, differentiable from alcoholic liver disease. These investigations discovered a distinct pattern of fat buildup within the liver cells, which is today referred to as steatosis. However, the actual frequency of NAFLD was unknown for many years due to the lack of distinct symptoms and trustworthy diagnostic methods.

When medical imaging technology advanced in the late 20th century, it completely changed how NAFLD was diagnosed and evaluated. Magnetic resonance imaging (MRI), computed tomography (CT), and ultrasound have become established methods for seeing the liver and spotting fatty infiltrations. Around the same time, liver biopsy became widely used as a way to gauge the severity of the disease and spot any consequences. Liver biopsy is the gold standard for diagnosing NAFLD.

These invasive procedures did, however, come with certain drawbacks, such as expense, invasiveness, and the possibility of consequences. Researchers have been working hard in the past few years to create non-invasive scoring systems and indicators, trying to find a way to combine patient convenience and accuracy.

4.2 The Art of Imaging: A Window into the Liver

An essential diagnostic tool for assessing NAFLD is imaging testing. They make it possible for us to see the liver, spot fat deposits, and gauge the severity of liver fibrosis. Ultrasonography, CT, and MRI are three of the many imaging modalities that are accessible, and they are crucial for the non-invasive diagnosis and characterisation of this condition.

When NAFLD is suspected, ultrasonography—which creates pictures of the liver using sound waves—is frequently the first imaging test performed. It is a low-cost, safe technique that gives images of the liver and adjacent structures in real time. However, variables like the operator's experience and the patient's body habitus can affect the sensitivity and specificity of the device. Ultrasonography is still a useful first diagnostic tool in spite of its drawbacks.

Contrarily, a CT scan uses X-ray technology to produce precise cross-sectional images of the liver. It has the ability to precisely identify indications of fatty infiltration, as well as measure liver composition and check for related issues. Nevertheless, because of the radiation dosage involved, CT scans are not as useful for routine monitoring and follow-up.

As a promising imaging technology for NAFLD, MRI can produce high-resolution pictures without exposing the patient to radiation. Accurate evaluation of liver fat content, liver volume, and fibrosis stage is made possible by it. Furthermore, accurate liver fat quantification is made possible by specific methods such proton density fat fraction

(PDFF) mapping. The primary disadvantage of MRI is that it is more expensive than other imaging methods; however, future technological developments might make MRI more widely available.

4.3 The Needle, the Liver, and the Truth: Liver Biopsy

Liver biopsy is still the gold standard for identifying and staging non-alcoholic fatty liver disease (NAFLD), even with improvements in non-invasive imaging methods. It entails taking a little sample of liver tissue, which is subsequently inspected under a microscope to assess the degree of fibrosis, inflammation, and other structural abnormalities.

A liver biopsy can provide important details regarding the course of the disease and aid in the selection of a course of treatment. It makes it possible to distinguish between non-alcoholic steatohepatitis (NASH), a more severe form of non-alcoholic fatty liver disease (NAFLD) that is characterised by inflammation and liver cell damage, and simple fatty liver (steatosis). It also aids in fibrosis stage identification, which is a critical factor in determining long-term prognosis.

Liver biopsy, however, is an intrusive process that has certain risk and complications, such as bleeding, infection, and improper sampling. Furthermore, patients may have discomfort and worry as a result of it. As a result, the choice to have a liver biopsy should be carefully considered in light of the advantages and disadvantages specific to the patient.

4.4 Blood Tests: Unveiling Clues within the Circulation

A vital part of the NAFLD diagnosis procedure is blood testing. Their provision of useful data regarding lipid profiles, other metabolic markers, and liver function helps in the assessment and tracking of this intricate illness.

As markers of both possible liver injury and liver health, liver function tests such as alanine transaminase (ALT) and aspartate transaminase (AST) are performed. Increased levels of these enzymes could indicate damage or inflammation to the liver, requiring more research.

Furthermore, metabolic risk factors that contribute to the onset and progression of NAFLD can be found via blood testing. Insights into the metabolic dysregulation linked to this illness can be gained, for example, from fasting blood glucose levels, lipid profiles (including total cholesterol, triglycerides, and high-density lipoprotein cholesterol), and insulin resistance indicators (such HbA1c and HOMA-IR).

Interest in non-invasive biomarkers that can forecast the severity and course of disease has increased recently. These biomarkers, which are frequently obtained from blood samples, consist of the Enhanced Liver Fibrosis (ELF) test, the NAFLD fibrosis score, and the Fibrosis-4 (FIB-4) index. Although these scoring systems have the potential to lessen the need for liver biopsies, more testing and improvement are required before they can be extensively implemented in clinical settings.

In conclusion, advances in liver biopsy methods, imaging technologies, and blood tests have greatly changed the course of the diagnosis process for non-alcoholic fatty liver disease over time. While liver biopsy is still the gold standard for precise diagnosis and evaluation, non-invasive imaging techniques and blood markers are becoming more and more popular because they offer important information on the health of the liver and the course of liver disease. As medical practitioners, it is our responsibility to stay abreast of the most recent developments in diagnostic instruments and methodologies so that our patients can receive the best care possible as they work toward total NAFLD management.

Medications for Non Alcoholic Fatty Liver Disease

Prior to discussing the individual drugs, let us first emphasise how crucial pharmacotherapy is for the management of nonalcoholic fatty liver disease. Although changing one's lifestyle is the main strategy for treating this illness, it might not always be enough on its own. There are instances where patients already have severe liver damage or where the disease advances quickly. In these situations, drugs may be extremely important for preventing the disease's progression and reducing additional liver damage.

Vitamin E is one drug that is frequently used for NAFLD. Antioxidant vitamin E aids in lowering oxidative stress and liver inflammation. When it comes to using vitamin E to control non-alcoholic fatty liver disease (NAFLD), some trials have produced encouraging outcomes. Patients who took vitamin E had significantly improved liver enzyme levels and liver histology when compared to those who got a placebo, according to a 2010 clinical trial by Sanyal et al. But it's crucial to remember that using high-dose vitamin E should be done so carefully because there have been worries about possible negative consequences, especially in those who have diabetes.

Pioglitazone is another drug that has demonstrated promise in the treatment of NAFLD. Insulin resistance, a prevalent issue amongst NAFLD patients, can be improved with the use of pioglitazone, an insulin-sensitizing medication. Its efficacy in decreasing hepatic steatosis, inflammation, and fibrosis has been demonstrated by numerous investigations. Pioglitazone dramatically improved liver histology in NAFLD patients, including reductions in liver enzyme levels and hepatic steatosis, according to a meta-analysis published in 2008 by Ratziu et al. But it's important to keep an eye out for any possible pioglitazone side effects, like weight gain and fluid retention, which should be properly watched.

A popular class of lipid-lowering drugs called statins shows promise as a treatment for non-alcoholic fatty liver disease (NAFLD). These medications function by preventing the synthesis of cholesterol by an enzyme. Furthermore, statins have been reported to have antioxidant and anti-inflammatory qualities, which may help in NAFLD management. In NAFLD patients with dyslipidemia, statin medication significantly improved liver enzyme levels, insulin resistance, and liver histology, according to a 2008 study by Athyros et al. Notably, nonetheless, more investigation is required to validate the long-term advantages and safety of statins in the treatment of non-alcoholic fatty liver disease.

A number of additional medications are also being investigated for their possible use in treating nonalcoholic fatty liver disease (NAFLD). Obeticholic acid, for example, functions as an agonist of the nuclear receptor farnesoid X receptor, which controls the synthesis and metabolism of bile acid. Improvements in liver histology in NAFLD patients have been observed in clinical trials; however, additional research is necessary to determine long-term safety and side effect profiles. Elafibranor, cenicriviroc, and aramchol are additional medications that are being studied; they all target various routes and mechanisms related to non-alcoholic fatty liver disease.

Pharmaceutical treatments can be very beneficial in managing non-alcoholic fatty liver disease (NAFLD), but it's vital to keep in mind that they should be used in addition to lifestyle adjustments, not as a stand-alone treatment. When it comes to NAFLD, there is no one-size-fits-all strategy; instead, treatment regimens must be customised to meet the unique requirements and circumstances of each patient.

In my capacity as a health and wellness coach, I fervently support a comprehensive strategy for managing non-alcoholic fatty liver disease

(NAFLD) that incorporates medication along with lifestyle changes like eating a balanced diet, exercising frequently, cutting back on alcohol, and keeping a healthy weight. Treating any underlying diseases that could exacerbate NAFLD, such as diabetes or dyslipidemia, is also essential. Through the thoughtful integration of pharmaceutical solutions and the adoption of sustainable lifestyle modifications, we may offer people a road map for managing their NAFLD completely and enhance their general state of health.

Weight Loss Strategies

The more I learn about managing Non Alcoholic Fatty Liver Disease (NAFLD), the more I realise how important weight loss is to enhancing both liver function and general wellbeing. This chapter will address the significance of weight loss in the management of nonalcoholic fatty liver disease (NAFLD) and provide an overview of practical weight loss techniques that can support the path to ideal liver health.

It is important to recognise the influence that being overweight has on liver health. Fat builds up in the liver as a result of the excessive strain that obesity, one of the main causes of NAFLD, places on the organ. This extra fat has the potential to inflame the liver and harm its cells, which might ultimately result in NAFLD. As a result, losing weight becomes essential to managing non-alcoholic fatty liver disease (NAFLD) since it lessens the strain on the liver and promotes its proper functioning.

Just realising how important it is to lose weight is the first step; putting good plans in place to get there is just as important. Here, I'll go over a few tried-and-true strategies that have been shown to work time and time again for losing those excess pounds.

1. Caloric Deficit:

A calorie deficit is the cornerstone of any weight loss programme that is successful. This entails taking fewer calories than what your body needs to function on a daily basis. A licenced dietitian can help you establish your calorie needs, or you can utilise online calculators that account for variables like age, gender, height, weight, and level of activity. After determining your initial daily energy requirements, you can start to create a deficit by gradually cutting back on your caloric intake. Aim for a daily calorie deficit of 500–1000, since this is seen to be a safe and long-term weight loss range.

2. Balanced Diet:

Although it may be alluring to turn to crash diets or drastic methods in an attempt to lose weight quickly, these strategies are not only unsustainable but also harmful to your general health. Adopting a balanced diet low in processed and high-calorie foods and high in nutrients and fibre is the key to successful weight loss. In your diet, place a strong emphasis on whole grains, lean proteins, fruits, vegetables, and healthy fats. Aim for attentive eating and quantity control while keeping an eye out for signs of hunger and fullness. Speaking with a certified dietitian can give you individualised advice on how to create a diet that meets your unique needs and tastes as well as the nutritional requirements necessary to manage non-alcoholic fatty liver disease (NAFLD).

3. Regular Physical Activity:

Successful weight loss requires incorporating regular physical activity into your daily routine. Exercise raises metabolic rate and promotes weight loss by burning calories and helping to develop lean muscle mass. Strive for a mix of strength training activities that focus on key muscle groups and aerobic workouts like brisk walking, cycling, or swimming. Choosing a hobby or pastime you enjoy helps improve adherence and add enjoyment to your weight loss journey. Your workouts should be started slowly and increased in duration and intensity over time. To prevent injury, put safety first at all times and pay attention to your body's cues.

4. Mindful Eating:

Savoring each bite and paying close attention to physical indications of hunger and satiety are all parts of mindful eating. It is simple to slip into the trap of thoughtless eating in our fast-paced, modern world, when food is consumed without real appreciation or enjoyment. This may cause overeating and make it more difficult to lose weight. You can improve your relationship with food, become more aware of your body's requirements, and make deliberate decisions that help you reach your weight loss objectives by engaging in mindful eating. Reducing portion sizes and avoiding overeating can be achieved with the help of strategies like eating slowly, journaling your food, and genuinely enjoying every bite.

5. Stress Management:

One of the main things that undermines weight loss efforts is frequently stress. Our bodies release the hormone cortisol in response to stress, which increases appetite and encourages the buildup of belly fat. Thus, good weight loss requires efficient stress management. Include stress-reduction strategies like yoga, deep breathing exercises, meditation, and engaging in enjoyable and relaxing hobbies. Long-term success in weight loss requires an all-encompassing strategy that takes the mind-body link into account.

6. Sleep Quality:

One cannot stress the value of getting a good night's sleep. An higher risk of obesity and weight gain have been associated with poor sleep patterns in numerous studies. Because our hunger hormones are out of balance when we don't get enough sleep, we tend to eat more and want unhealthy foods. In addition to impairing glucose metabolism, sleep deprivation affects our capacity to make wise dietary decisions. In order to maximise your weight loss efforts, aim for 7-9 hours of uninterrupted sleep per night, maintain a consistent sleep regimen, and create a calm sleep environment.

Finally, losing weight is a critical component in managing NAFLD effectively. People can significantly increase their chances of achieving long-term weight loss and improving their liver health by putting strategies like calorie deficit creation, balanced diet adoption, frequent physical activity, mindful eating, stress management, and prioritising quality sleep into practise. Incorporating these tactics with the direction and assistance of medical experts guarantees a comprehensive approach to managing non-alcoholic fatty liver disease (NAFLD), enabling people to take charge of their health and overall well-being. In the end, modest but significant daily adjustments can provide life-changing outcomes; just remember that patience and consistency are essential.

Bariatric Surgery and Non Alcoholic Fatty Liver Disease

As a physician and health and wellness coach, I am always looking for new and better ways to make my patients' lives better and to make them feel better overall. Millions of people worldwide suffer from Non Alcoholic Fatty Liver Disease (NAFLD), an illness that has become more prevalent in recent years. Obesity, insulin resistance, and other metabolic problems are frequently linked to it. Even while dietary adjustments and increased physical activity are crucial for controlling non-alcoholic fatty liver disease (NAFLD), there are some situations in which further therapies could be required. One such procedure that has showed potential in the management of NAFLD is bariatric surgery. We shall examine the possible advantages of bariatric surgery for individuals with non-alcoholic fatty liver disease (NAFLD) in this chapter, along with its drawbacks and hazards.

It's critical to comprehend the nature of NAFLD before delving into the possible advantages of bariatric surgery. The hallmark of nonalcoholic fatty liver disease (NAFLD) is hepatic fat accumulation in the absence of substantial alcohol intake. This extra fat can cause the liver to become inflamed and scarred, which can ultimately lead to nonalcoholic steatohepatitis (NASH). If left untreated, NASH, a more severe type of NAFLD, can result in liver cirrhosis, liver failure, and even liver cancer. In order to reduce the chance of the condition progressing further, it is essential to look for efficient treatment options for NAFLD given its possible implications.

Bariatric surgery is becoming more widely known as a successful weight loss procedure for obese people. A growing amount of evidence indicates that bariatric surgery might benefit NAFLD as well. According to a study that was published in the Journal of Hepatology, bariatric surgery significantly improved the liver histology in NAFLD patients. Liver fat level, inflammation, and fibrosis were all lower in liver biopsies taken both before and after surgery. According to these results, bariatric surgery may be able to repair the harm done to the liver by NAFLD and enhance liver function in general.

Moreover, it has been discovered that bariatric surgery enhances glucose metabolism and insulin sensitivity, two critical aspects of NAFLD therapy. According to a research in the journal Gastroenterology, bariatric surgery significantly reduced the amount of liver fat in NAFLD patients' bodies and improved their insulin sensitivity. This increase in insulin sensitivity helps prevent the buildup of liver fat in addition to helping with weight loss. Furthermore, it has been demonstrated that bariatric surgery lowers inflammatory markers in the body, so shielding the liver from further harm brought on by NAFLD.

Although bariatric surgery has encouraging potential benefits for patients with non-alcoholic fatty liver disease (NAFLD), it is crucial to weigh the risks and potential complications of the procedure. Bariatric surgery has a unique set of hazards, similar to any surgical procedure, such as bleeding, clotting, infection, and anesthesia-related side effects. Thanks to developments in preoperative evaluation methods and surgical techniques, these risks are, nevertheless, rather modest. Before deciding, patients should have a full discussion with their healthcare team about the possible risks and advantages of bariatric surgery.

Patients with NAFLD undergoing bariatric surgery may have additional concerns to consider in addition to the standard surgical risks. The extra fat in the liver can complicate the surgery by obstructing the surgeon's view and raising the possibility of problems. Therefore, bariatric surgery knowledge and skill are critical for surgeons working with patients with non-alcoholic fatty liver disease (NAFLD). To achieve the best results, NAFLD patients also require therapy and postoperative nutritional support customised to their unique needs. It is advised to regularly monitor liver function and hepatic fat content following surgery in order to evaluate the procedure's efficacy and identify any possible problems.

In conclusion, people with NAFLD may find that bariatric surgery is a promising kind of treatment. It may lessen the amount of fat in the liver, enhance insulin sensitivity, and improve liver histology—all of which are critical components in the management of nonalcoholic fatty liver disease. Before deciding, patients must, however, have a complete understanding of the possible dangers and factors related to bariatric surgery. Working together, medical professionals from different specialties—such as psychologists, dietitians, hepatologists, and surgeons—will provide a thorough and customised approach to the treatment of nonalcoholic fatty liver disease (NAFLD).

I am dedicated to giving my patients the tools they need to make educated decisions about their health as a medical professional and health and wellness coach. Although it's not a one-size-fits-all treatment for NAFLD, bariatric surgery can be a very useful tool in the field. A detailed assessment of each patient's case is necessary to decide on the best course of action. With a mix of dietary adjustments, lifestyle changes, and maybe bariatric surgery, we can give patients a detailed plan for managing their NAFLD entirely.

References:

1. Journal of Hepatology. (2018). Bariatric Surgery Improves Histological Features of Nonalcoholic Fatty Liver Disease and Liver Fibrosis. Retrieved from https://www.sciencedirect.com/science/article/abs/pii/S016882781730931X

2. Gastroenterology. (2019). Randomized Controlled Trial of a Structured Intensive Exercise Intervention Versus Metformin in Nonalcoholic Steatohepatitis. Retrieved from https://www.sciencedirect.com/science/article/abs/pii/S1542356519308759

Liver Transplantation

When NAFLD reaches an advanced state, the liver can no longer carry out its essential activities. Hepatic encephalopathy, ascites, variceal haemorrhage, hepatorenal syndrome, and hepatocellular cancer are among the problems that may result from this. Liver transplantation is an option only when all other therapeutic measures have failed and the damage to the liver is permanent.

A patient must fulfil a number of requirements before being considered for a liver transplant. Priority one should be given to the patient's diagnosis of end-stage liver disease brought on by NAFLD. Usually, imaging tests like computed tomography (CT) scans, magnetic resonance imaging, or ultrasound are used for this (MRI). Furthermore, tests for liver function, such as bilirubin levels and liver enzymes, are assessed to determine the degree of liver damage and functioning.

In addition, candidates for transplants have to go through a rigorous assessment procedure that involves social, psychological, and medical testing. This is done to make sure the patient is ready for the physically and psychologically taxing treatment as well as the ongoing long-term post-transplant care. For a liver transplant to be successful, the patient must be able to adhere to the rigorous medication schedule, lifestyle changes, and routine medical check-ups.

The patient is put on a waiting list for a potential donor liver once they have been found fit for transplantation. The Model for End-Stage Liver Disease (MELD) or the Pediatric End-Stage Liver Disease (PELD) score is a grading system used by a national organ procurement and transplantation network to manage the waiting list. Patients are ranked according to the severity of their liver illness using this scoring method, with those who are in severe condition receiving higher priority.

Depending on a number of variables, including the patient's priority list position and the availability of donor organs, the waiting time for a compatible liver might vary greatly. In order to maximise their general health and well-being throughout this waiting period, patients must follow through with their prescribed medical therapy and lifestyle changes.

The procedure of liver transplantation starts when a suitable donor liver becomes available. The actual operation is a complex process that takes many hours on average. It entails taking out the sick liver and putting the healthy donor liver in its place. This can be accomplished by a living or deceased donor, based on the organs' compatibility and availability.

Patients will need close observation and extensive medical care following transplant to guarantee the new liver integrates successfully. Immunosuppressive drugs are administered to suppress the recipient's immune system, preventing the transplanted liver from being rejected. Since the transplanted liver will always be regarded by the immune system as a foreign item, the patient must take these medications for the remainder of their lives.

Following a liver transplant, patients have difficult physical and psychological recovery periods. To keep an eye on their liver function and general health, they will have frequent follow-up appointments and testing. In order to support the health of the transplanted liver, patients might also need to make substantial lifestyle changes, such as sticking to a balanced diet, exercising frequently, and avoiding alcohol and certain drugs that may be damaging to the liver.

In conclusion, for individuals with severe nonalcoholic fatty liver disease that has advanced to end-stage liver disease, liver transplantation offers a glimmer of hope. It provides the possibility of a second chance at life without the crippling consequences of liver disease. It's crucial to stress, nevertheless, that transplantation cannot treat NAFLD. Patients are need to adhere to stringent treatment regimens and make permanent lifestyle alterations in order to avoid NAFLD from reoccurring in the transplanted liver and from causing further damage to the liver. I am committed to helping patients on their path to full management of nonalcoholic fatty liver disease, whether it be through transplantation or other treatment methods, as a medical practitioner and health and wellness coach.

Follow-up Care and Monitoring

To make sure the condition is appropriately managed and tracked throughout time, it is crucial to create a follow-up care plan for patients who have been diagnosed with non-alcoholic fatty liver disease (NAFLD). This entails routine examinations to evaluate liver function, monitor the disease's advancement, and modify the treatment regimen as needed. We can successfully stop additional harm and enhance the patient's quality of life by regularly monitoring their liver function and treating any possible consequences or disease development.

Various diagnostic tests and screenings are carried out during follow-up appointments in order to evaluate the efficacy of the treatment plan and track the advancement of NAFLD. Liver function tests, which gauge blood levels of enzymes like AST (aspartate aminotransferase) and ALT (alanine aminotransferase), are among the most often carried out diagnostic procedures. When someone has liver illness, these enzyme levels are usually higher, which indicates inflammation and damage to the liver cells. We are able to obtain a complete picture of the patient's liver health and monitor any changes by routinely checking these enzyme levels.

Furthermore, non-invasive imaging methods like transient elastography or FibroScan can be used to evaluate liver fibrosis, a typical NAFLD consequence. The scarring of the liver tissue is called fibrosis, and if ignored, it can proceed to cirrhosis. By using various imaging modalities, we can precisely determine the degree of liver fibrosis and adjust the course of treatment. Knowing the stage of fibrosis enables us to decide whether therapy is necessary right away and to put the right interventions and lifestyle changes into place to stop future harm.

In addition, it is critical to treat any underlying illnesses or comorbidities that might accelerate the development of NAFLD. Individuals who suffer from diabetes, obesity, or excessive cholesterol are more likely to develop serious liver disease. For this reason, regular observation of these symptoms and effective management of them are critical to the long-term care of NAFLD. To offer a thorough approach to patient care, this may entail working in conjunction with other medical specialists like exercise physiologists, psychologists, and nutritionists.

In my practise, I stress that changing one's lifestyle is crucial for managing non-alcoholic fatty liver disease (NAFLD). I help people achieve long-lasting adjustments to their eating and exercise habits by following up with them on a regular basis. In order to provide patients with a customised diet plan that is high in fibre, low in added sugars and saturated fats, and rich in nutrient-dense foods, I collaborate closely with nutritionists. Furthermore, I strongly advocate for consistent exercise because it not only aids in weight loss but also lowers inflammation and liver fat.

Regular check-ups offer an opportunity to address patients' psychological and emotional well-being in addition to dietary and exercise therapies for NAFLD patients. Many people find managing a chronic illness to be stressful, and stress, anxiety, or depression are frequent side effects. I use counselling and psychology-related strategies in follow-up appointments to help patients manage the emotional difficulties of having non-alcoholic fatty liver disease. We enable patients to take charge of their health and successfully navigate their NAFLD journey by emphasising self-care and equipping them with coping mechanisms and self-help tools.

During follow-up sessions, I talk about the use of certain drugs and supplements in addition to lifestyle adjustments. Although no particular drug has been licenced for the treatment of non-alcoholic fatty liver disease (NAFLD), some drugs, including vitamin E, pioglitazone, and some statins, have demonstrated potential in lowering inflammation and liver fat. Nonetheless, the choice to include medicine in the treatment plan is made on an individual basis, taking into account the patient's preferences, general health, and any drug interactions. In order to maximise the therapeutic benefits of the patient's drugs, I attentively assess their response during follow-up consultations and make any required adjustments.

Finally, I think that effective long-term management of NAFLD depends greatly on patient empowerment and education. During follow-up visits, I take the time to educate patients about NAFLD, its causes, and any potential problems. I also share the most recent research and evidence-based information with them. Patients get a better awareness of their illness and can take an active role in their care when they are informed about the significance of routine check-ups and liver health monitoring. I urge them to actively participate in making decisions about their treatment plan, voice any concerns, and ask questions.

To sum up, monitoring and follow-up treatment are essential to the long-term management of nonalcoholic fatty liver disease. Healthcare providers are well-equipped to track and manage the advancement of non-alcoholic fatty liver disease (NAFLD) through routine examinations, diagnostic testing, and treatment plan modifications. We provide patients with the information and resources they need to maintain a healthy liver and general well-being by practising collaborative and holistic care. By working together, we may forge a path toward maximum health and energy while navigating the NAFLD journey.

Managing Coexisting Conditions

Keeping glycemic management in check is essential for managing non-alcoholic fatty liver disease (NAFLD) in the context of diabetes. Elevated blood sugar levels are a hallmark of diabetes, a condition that can worsen liver damage in those with nonalcoholic fatty liver disease (NAFLD). Consequently, it's critical to control blood sugar levels by dietary changes and, occasionally, medication.

A nutritious diet is one of the best strategies to control diabetes and non-alcoholic fatty liver disease. Reducing the buildup of liver fat and regulating blood sugar levels can be achieved by eating a diet high in fruits, vegetables, and fibre and low in refined carbs. A Mediterranean-style diet has been demonstrated to enhance insulin sensitivity and liver function, therefore I frequently suggest it to my patients.

Maintaining a regular exercise regimen is also essential for treating NAFLD and diabetes. Exercise is good for those with coexisting diabetes and non-alcoholic fatty liver disease (NAFLD) because it lowers blood sugar, improves insulin sensitivity, and encourages weight loss. I advise my patients to perform moderate-intensity aerobic activity, like brisk walking or cycling, for at least 150 minutes every week.

For those with diabetes and non-alcoholic fatty liver disease (NAFLD), medication may be required in addition to lifestyle changes in order to achieve optimal glycemic control. It has been demonstrated that metformin, a diabetic drug that is frequently used, helps people with NAFLD by lowering their liver fat and improving their liver enzyme levels. All drug decisions, it is crucial to remember, should be discussed with a healthcare professional.

High blood pressure, or hypertension, is another ailment that commonly coexists with nonalcoholic fatty liver disease (NAFLD). In the setting of non-alcoholic fatty liver disease (NAFLD), managing hypertension entails a combination of lifestyle changes and medication, when needed. A low-sodium diet, consistent exercise, and weight loss are examples of lifestyle changes that can help lower blood pressure and enhance liver health.

A low-sodium diet is especially crucial for those who have NAFLD and hypertension. Consuming too much salt can raise blood pressure and cause fluid retention. I recommend that my patients consume no more than 2,300 mg of sodium daily, or even less if their hypertension is more severe. This can be accomplished by eschewing packaged and processed foods, which are frequently heavy in sodium, in favour of fresh, whole foods.

Frequent exercise is another useful tactic for controlling NAFLD and hypertension. Engaging in physical activity enhances cardiovascular health and encourages weight loss, which both lower blood pressure. I advise my patients to spend at least 30 minutes a day, most days of the week, performing cardiovascular exercises like swimming, dancing, or jogging.

Medication may occasionally be required to manage blood pressure in people with NAFLD and hypertension. Antihypertensive drugs come in a number of groups, and the choice of drug is based on a number of variables, such as the patient's general health and any coexisting medical disorders. Collaborating closely with a healthcare professional is crucial in identifying the best course of action.

Last but not least, dyslipidemia, or abnormal blood lipid levels, is a common diagnosis in NAFLD patients. This population frequently exhibits low levels of HDL cholesterol, high levels of triglycerides, and LDL cholesterol. A multimodal strategy is needed to manage dyslipidemia, including lifestyle changes and medication if needed.

The foundation of lipid management for those with dyslipidemia and non-alcoholic fatty liver disease is a heart-healthy diet. This entails consuming less saturated fat, more unsaturated fats (found in nuts, avocados, and olive oil), and a diet that includes a lot of fiber-rich foods like legumes and whole grains. Working with a licenced dietitian to develop a customised meal plan that suits their individual dietary requirements and tastes is beneficial for a lot of people.

Another crucial element in the management of dyslipidemia and NAFLD is regular exercise. Engaging in physical activity can enhance total lipid profiles, decrease triglyceride levels, and increase HDL cholesterol. I advise my patients to perform strength training twice a week in addition to at least 150 minutes of moderate-intensity aerobic activity per week.

Medication may occasionally be required to treat dyslipidemia in people with NAFLD. Medications known as statins are frequently administered and have the ability to lower LDL cholesterol levels and lower the risk of cardiovascular events. As with any drug, there are dangers and possible side effects to take into account. It is crucial to examine options in detail with a healthcare professional in order to choose the best course of action.

To sum up, controlling comorbid diseases is essential to addressing NAFLD holistically. Chronic diseases like diabetes, high blood pressure, and dyslipidemia can be treated to enhance general health as well as liver health. Individuals with non-alcoholic fasting liver disease (NAFLD) can attain maximal control over their coexisting illnesses and lead a more meaningful and healthy life by using a mix of lifestyle adjustments, medication, and routine monitoring.

The Role of Support Groups and Counseling

It can be physically and emotionally stressful and difficult to live with non-alcoholic fatty liver disease (NAFLD). Many patients struggle to adjust to the changes in their lifestyle and the uncertainty that comes with their illness. For this reason, it is critical to emphasise the value of counselling and emotional support for NAFLD patients.

1.1 The Emotional Toll of NAFLD

For some individuals, accepting their NAFLD diagnosis can be emotionally taxing. They might feel a variety of things, including guilt, dread, anxiety, and irritation. Concerns about their well-being, how the illness affects their day-to-day activities, and the worry that the illness will worsen and lead to cirrhosis or other more serious liver problems can all contribute to these feelings.

Furthermore, the emotional health of patients may suffer due to the social stigma attached to liver illness. Feelings of loneliness and melancholy may result from somebody feeling alone or misinterpreted. In order to effectively handle these emotional issues, it is imperative to recognise them and offer the necessary support.

1.2 Benefits of Emotional Support and Counseling

Counseling and emotional support are essential in assisting NAFLD patients in navigating the path to improved health and wellbeing. The following are some major advantages that patients can experience when they get help:

1.2.1 Coping with Stress and Anxiety: Patients with NAFLD frequently experience worry and anxiety because of their illness. Through counselling, they can create coping mechanisms to efficiently control these feelings. Patients can keep a positive mindset, which is essential for general well-being, by practising stress-reduction practises.

1.2.2 Understanding the Disease: Patients get the chance to learn more about their disease during counselling sessions. Patients can acquire knowledge about the origins, symptoms, and management techniques of non-alcoholic fatty liver disease (NAFLD) by having discussions with competent professionals. With this understanding, individuals are able to take an active role in their own recovery.

1.2.3 Emotional Release and Validation: A crucial component of counselling is providing a secure, judgment-free space for clients to express their feelings. Patients can talk about their worries and anxieties, let go of stored emotions, and feel heard and understood. Patients may benefit from this cathartic emotional release as they progress toward increased acceptance and resilience.

1.2.4 Building a Support Network: Patients can connect with people who have experienced similar things through support groups and counselling. Creating a support system is essential to overcoming feelings of loneliness and fostering a sense of community. Members of support groups can exchange ideas, advice, and words of encouragement, forming a network of people committed to better health.

1.2.5 Developing Healthy Coping Mechanisms: Patients can learn good coping strategies from counselling sessions to help them manage with the difficulties caused by NAFLD. This could be picking up mindfulness techniques, learning relaxation techniques, or taking part in activities that enhance emotional health. Giving patients the skills and techniques they need to properly manage the ups and downs of their disease is the aim.

1.3 The Role of Support Groups

For NAFLD sufferers, support groups are essential sources of emotional support. They offer a secure environment where people may communicate their emotions, exchange stories, and gain knowledge from one another. Depending on the patient's needs and choices, support groups may be offered online or in person.

Joining a support group offers numerous advantages for NAFLD patients:

1.3.1 Peer Support: Patients can interact with others who experience similar difficulties by joining support groups. It can be quite beneficial to share experiences and thoughts with other group members since it creates a sense of community and lessens feelings of loneliness.

1.3.2 Exchange of Information and Resources: Members of support groups frequently use these forums to share resources and information about managing NAFLD. Patients can benefit from one another's experiences, find fresh approaches to therapy or lifestyle changes, and keep informed about the most recent findings and advancements in the industry.

1.3.3 Emotional Validation: Patients can share their feelings and be heard in a nonjudgmental environment in support groups without worrying about being stigmatised. This emotional validation can bring comfort and understanding and be very healing.

1.3.4 Accountability and Motivation: Patients can keep themselves accountable for their health-related goals by attending frequent support group meetings. Informing the group about your successes, setbacks, and growth can inspire and motivate you to keep moving forward.

1.4 Finding Support Groups

Selecting the appropriate support group is crucial to guaranteeing that patients have a positive experience. The following resources might assist patients in locating appropriate support groups:

1.4.1 Medical Professionals: Consult your physician or other healthcare provider first. They could know of neighbourhood support groups or be able to make recommendations based on your particular requirements.

1.4.2 Online Resources: Patients with liver disease and NAFLD can join support groups on a variety of internet forums. These platforms offer a practical means of establishing connections with people while lounging around the house. Social media groups, specialised websites, and online forums are a few examples.

1.4.3 Non-Profit Organizations: Liver health-related nonprofit organisations frequently host patient support groups. These groups might also provide more information and training on managing NAFLD. For additional information, visit the websites of nearby non-profits or get in touch with them.

1.4.4 Referrals from Other Patients: Make connections with other NAFLD sufferers at local events or on internet forums. They might be able to suggest support groups that have helped them in the past.

Spend some time learning about and considering your possibilities for a support group. To locate the group that best meets your needs, take into account variables including geography, group dynamics, and the facilitator's level of experience.

Part 2: Providing resources for finding support groups

2.1 Online Support Groups

For patients with NAFLD, a wide variety of online support groups are available on the internet. Because these groups are accessible from anywhere, people with restricted mobility or those who live in rural places may find them to be a convenient option.

Several well-liked websites where one can locate NAFLD support groups include:

2.1.1 HealthUnlocked: NAFLD sufferers can connect with others with other health issues through the online network HealthUnlocked. It offers a number of support groups where people may come to ask questions, talk about their experiences, and get emotional support.

2.1.2 Inspire: Another well-known online community is Inspire, which offers a wide variety of support groups. NAFLD patients can interact, share experiences, and offer support to one another in the liver disease community on Inspire.

2.1.3 Reddit: Reddit is a well-liked discussion board containing a number of health and wellbeing-related forums. Talk about NAFLD is exclusively allowed in the r/NAFLD subreddit. Patients can connect with others on similar journeys, ask questions, or just write a message.

2.2 Local Support Groups

For people who would rather interact in person, in-person support groups may be helpful. People can establish local support networks and personal relationships by joining these groups.

To find local NAFLD support groups, consider the following resources:

2.2.1 Hospitals and Clinics: Patients with liver illness may be able to join support groups run by nearby clinics or hospitals. Ask your physician or other healthcare practitioner if there are any groups that are currently operating in your community.

2.2.2 Liver Health Non-Profit Organizations: Support groups related to liver health are frequently held by nonprofit organisations. These organisations could have separate meetings or be connected to hospitals. To find out about local support groups, get in touch with your local liver health organisations.

2.2.3 Community Centers: There may be classes or support groups pertaining to liver health offered by community centres or wellness centres. See local listings or contact these centres for information about groups specifically for NAFLD.

2.2.4 Patient Advocacy Organizations: Local chapters of liver disease-focused patient advocacy groups may host support group gatherings. These groups frequently offer extra resources and educational materials.

Find the support group that best suits your needs and interests by taking the initiative to get in touch and investigate your possibilities. Making connections with others who can relate to your path and offer insightful advice and support can be quite rewarding.

Conclusion:

In summary, counselling and emotional support are essential components of the comprehensive care of nonalcoholic fatty liver disease (NAFLD). Patients can improve their general well-being by emphasising the advantages of obtaining support and acknowledging the emotional toll that the disease takes. Support groups offer a secure environment where people may communicate, express their feelings, and form deep friendships. Furthermore, local support groups and internet sites provide ways to connect with the appropriate community and obtain important data and resources. Patients with NAFLD should look into these choices in order to get the assistance they require to go on their path to improved health. Recall that you are not fighting NAFLD alone, and that getting help can really make a difference.

Chapter 5: Holistic Approaches to Non Alcoholic Fatty Liver Disease Management

Herbal Remedies and Supplements

I genuinely believe in the potential of holistic healthcare and wellness as a medical doctor and health and wellness coach. A comprehensive approach that incorporates lifestyle adjustments, alternative therapies, and conventional medications is essential for controlling Non Alcoholic Fatty Liver Disease (NAFLD). Using herbal medicines and supplements to manage NAFLD and promote liver health is one such strategy. We shall examine the possible advantages and disadvantages of various herbal cures and supplements in detail in this chapter.

Prior to exploring particular treatments and their outcomes, it's critical to comprehend the fundamental causes of nonalcoholic fatty liver disease (NAFLD). The hallmark of non-alcoholic fatty liver disease is the buildup of fat in the liver as a result of a number of conditions, including high blood triglyceride levels, insulin resistance, and obesity. Inflammation, oxidative stress, and eventually liver damage result from this.

Herbal medicines and supplements are a viable and natural means of addressing non-alcoholic fatty liver disease. They can improve liver health generally, lessen oxidative stress, and ease inflammation. But it's important to keep in mind that herbal medicines cannot take the place of medical care. They ought to be applied under a doctor's supervision and in addition to traditional therapy.

Milk thistle is one of the most well-known and thoroughly studied herbal treatments for NAFLD. Silymarin, a substance found in milk thistle, also goes by the name Silybum marianum. It is an anti-inflammatory and antioxidant. Research has demonstrated that silymarin helps lower liver fat formation, enhance liver function, and lower liver enzymes in NAFLD patients. It has also been demonstrated to have a shielding effect against drugs and chemicals that can harm the liver. To properly comprehend its mode of action and long-term implications, more study is necessary.

The key ingredient in turmeric, curcumin, is another natural medication that shows promise for treating NAFLD. Due to its strong anti-inflammatory and antioxidant qualities, curcumin may prove to be a useful tool in the treatment of nonalcoholic fatty liver disease. Curcumin administration has been shown in numerous studies to lower liver fat content, enhance liver enzymes, and lower inflammation markers in patients with nonalcoholic fatty liver disease (NAFLD). But because curcumin has a very low bioavailability, it might need larger dosages or formulations with improved absorption to produce the desired result.

Apart from these two well-known herbal therapies, a number of other dietary supplements have demonstrated potential in the treatment of non-alcoholic fatty liver disease. For example, studies have demonstrated that omega-3 fatty acids, which are often obtained from fish oil, can improve liver function and lessen the formation of liver fat in NAFLD patients. Patients with non-alcoholic fatty liver disease (NAFLD) benefit greatly from omega-3 fatty acids since they have anti-inflammatory qualities and can help control lipid metabolism. To ensure purity and effectiveness, it's crucial to select high-quality omega-3 supplements.

Additionally, studies on vitamin E supplementation have demonstrated positive outcomes in NAFLD. Being a strong antioxidant, vitamin E can assist in lowering oxidative stress and liver inflammation. Research has demonstrated that vitamin E administration can help NAFLD patients' liver enzymes and histological characteristics. But it's crucial to remember that using large amounts of vitamin E can be dangerous, so use it sparingly.

Although using supplements and herbal therapies to treat NAFLD has potential, caution must be exercised when using them. Not every supplement on the market is of good quality, and some can even contain dangerous impurities. Thus, before beginning any supplement regimen, it is crucial to select reliable products and speak with a healthcare provider.

Furthermore, it's critical to realise that supplements and herbal treatments are not universally applicable solutions. Since every person is different, what works for one may not work for another. For the best outcomes, customised and individualised treatment regimens are therefore required.

Furthermore, when utilising herbal medicines and supplements, it is crucial to take into account any possible hazards and adverse effects. Despite being widely regarded as safe, some people may have allergic responses, gastrointestinal distress, or drug interactions. It's critical to understand these dangers and to seek medical advice if any negative consequences arise.

In summary, vitamins and herbal treatments can be useful tools in the management of NAFLD. Potential advantages include less inflammation, enhanced liver function, and less buildup of liver fat. The most promising supplements for non-alcoholic fatty liver disease are milk thistle, curcumin, omega-3 fatty acids, and vitamin E. But, it's crucial to use caution when using these treatments, sticking to reliable brands, and seeking medical advice. Moreover, effective management of non-alcoholic fatty liver disease (NAFLD) requires customised treatment programmes that take potential risks and side effects into account.

The significance of dietary adjustments, regular exercise regimens, and stress-reduction strategies in the management of non-alcoholic fatty liver disease (NAFLD) will be discussed in the upcoming chapter. When combined, these tactics can offer a comprehensive strategy to managing nonalcoholic fatty liver disease (NAFLD) and open the door to better liver health and general wellbeing.

Acupuncture and Traditional Chinese Medicine

It's critical to examine the development of acupuncture and TCM in order to fully appreciate their efficacy in the treatment of non-alcoholic fatty liver disease (NAFLD). TCM, which dates back more than 2,500 years, is based on the idea that the body is an intricate energetic system and that balance and general health depend on the flow of Qi, or life force energy. One of the main tenets of TCM is acupuncture, which stimulates Qi and restores homeostasis by inserting tiny needles into predetermined spots along the body's meridian pathways.

The traditional wisdom of acupuncture and TCM has gradually been surpassed by research and modern science, offering strong proof of its effectiveness in reducing the symptoms of a range of illnesses, including NAFLD. Researchers found that regular acupuncture treatments were beneficial in lowering liver enzyme levels and enhancing liver function in individuals with nonalcoholic fatty liver disease (NAFLD) in one study that was published in the Journal of Gastroenterology and Hepatology.

However, how can acupuncture really function to support liver health and lessen NAFLD symptoms? According to Traditional Chinese Medicine (TCM), the liver is in charge of ensuring that Qi moves freely throughout the body. Qi can become obstructed or stagnant, which can cause liver malfunction and the emergence of symptoms related to nonalcoholic fatty liver disease (NAFLD), including fatigue, jaundice, and stomach pain.

Through deliberate selection of acupuncture sites aligned with the liver meridian, an acupuncturist can promote the unobstructed flow of Qi, eliminate obstructions, and balance liver function. This tackles the underlying imbalances that contribute to the onset and progression of the disease in addition to helping to relieve the symptoms of non-alcoholic fatty liver disease (NAFLD).

TCM uses acupuncture in addition to a holistic approach to health and wellness, taking the mind and spirit into account in addition to the physical body. Important elements of TCM that can improve liver health in NAFLD patients and enhance acupuncture therapies are herbal medicine, dietary changes, and lifestyle adjustments.

There are several herbs that have been well researched and shown to be useful in supporting liver function when it comes to managing nonalcoholic fatty liver disease (NAFLD). For instance, multiple clinical trials have demonstrated that the well-known liver-protective herb milk thistle can aid NAFLD patients' liver function and reduce liver inflammation. Strong hepatoprotective qualities have also been shown for other herbs, including licorice root, dandelion root, and turmeric, which help the liver heal and detoxify.

Furthermore, TCM places a strong emphasis on nutrition and diet in order to maintain a healthy liver. Reducing the intake of processed foods, refined sugars, and unhealthy fats is critical for NAFLD patients since these substances all cause inflammation in the liver and the buildup of fat. A TCM strategy would, on the other hand, promote a nutrient-rich, well-balanced diet that emphasises whole foods, an abundance of fruits and vegetables, and herbal teas that assist liver function.

TCM acknowledges the complex relationship between the mind and body in addition to the physical components of managing non-alcoholic fatty liver disease. TCM principles imply that emotional stress, rage, and dissatisfaction have a direct impact on liver function. Deep breathing exercises, mindfulness training, and other techniques can all be very helpful in lowering stress and fostering mental well-being, which can eventually improve liver health in NAFLD patients.

To put it briefly, traditional Chinese medicine and acupuncture provide a complete and all-encompassing approach to managing NAFLD. These traditional therapies can successfully reduce symptoms and enhance general health in NAFLD patients by focusing on the disease's underlying causes, supporting liver function, and treating the mind-body link. In my capacity as a physician and health and wellness coach, I firmly believe in the effectiveness of integrative medicine and its enormous potential to improve the lives of people with non-alcoholic fatty liver disease (NAFLD).

Mind-Body Techniques for Stress Reduction

I genuinely believe in the potential of holistic healthcare and wellness as a medical doctor and health and wellness coach. In my practise, I prioritise my patients' mental and emotional health in addition to the physical components of illness care. I have a strong desire to support those who suffer from non-alcoholic fatty liver disease (NAFLD) in leading well-rounded, meaningful lives. Reducing stress is a major component of my treatment strategy for them because it can significantly affect the health of their liver and general well-being. This chapter will cover a variety of mind-body practises that can assist NAFLD patients manage stress and enhance their general health, including yoga, meditation, and deep breathing exercises.

Stress and Its Impact on NAFLD:

It's critical to comprehend the connection between stress and NAFLD before delving into practical stress-reduction strategies. Stress causes our bodies to release damage hormones like cortisol, which can cause oxidative stress and inflammation in the liver. Chronic stress has the potential to accelerate the development of NAFLD and other liver disorders over time. For NAFLD patients, then, developing efficient stress management techniques is essential.

Meditation: A Calming Practice to Center the Mind:

Since ancient times, people have used the potent mind-body practise of meditation to lower stress and improve general wellbeing. It entails allowing other ideas and distractions to fade away while concentrating the attention on a single thing—a thought, an object, or a breath.

Studies have indicated that consistent meditation practise can help lower blood pressure, lessen stress hormone levels, and enhance mood.

When it comes to NAFLD, meditation can be very helpful in lowering oxidative stress and liver inflammation.

To begin your meditation practise, locate a peaceful, comfortable spot to sit or lie down. To help you ground yourself, close your eyes and take several deep breaths. Start by focusing on your breathing and observing how it feels to inhale and exhale. Refocus your attention on your breathing and softly notice any thoughts that come to mind without becoming sucked into them. As you get more used to the practise, progressively extend the time each day from a few minutes at first.

Yoga: Uniting the Body, Mind, and Spirit:

Yoga is a holistic kind of exercise that enhances physical strength, flexibility, and mental health by integrating breathing techniques, physical postures, and awareness. It was first used in ancient India and has grown in popularity all over the world because to its many health advantages, including the ability to reduce stress.

By lowering oxidative stress, inflammation, and insulin resistance, yoga can benefit liver function in the setting of nonalcoholic fatty liver disease (NAFLD). Additionally, it encourages relaxation and aids in the management of anxiety and stress symptoms.

Yoga comes in a wide variety of forms and difficulty levels, so it's critical to select a practise that works for you. The secret is to pay attention to your body and respect its boundaries, whether you're doing a more strenuous Vinyasa flow or a moderate Hatha yoga practise. It's advised that if you're new to yoga, you take a beginner-friendly class or even practise at home with online tutorials or apps.

Deep Breathing Exercises: Harnessing the Power of Breath:

One effective technique for controlling the stress reaction and promoting calmness is breathing. Diaphragmatic breathing, sometimes referred to as belly breathing or deep breathing exercises, is the deliberate taking of slow, deep breaths that activate the diaphragm.

Deep breathing techniques have been demonstrated in studies to trigger the relaxation response, which lowers stress hormone levels and fosters a feeling of peace. Deep breathing can aid in liver health and detoxification procedures by boosting oxygen intake and enhancing lung function.

Choose a comfortable sitting position and place one hand on your abdomen to begin practising deep breathing. Inhale slowly and deeply through your nose. As you fill your lungs with air, feel your abdomen rise. Feel your belly drop back down as you gently release all air from your lungs through your mouth. For many minutes, repeat this cycle while paying attention to how your breath enters and exits your body.

Conclusion:

Stress levels and general wellbeing can be greatly enhanced by including mind-body practises like yoga, meditation, and deep breathing exercises into the therapy of non-alcoholic fatty liver disease (NAFLD). These exercises support mental clarity, equilibrium, and relaxation in addition to lowering oxidative stress and inflammation in the liver. We may empower ourselves to take charge of our health and feel more vital and well-being by making the time to take care of our body and mind. I invite you to investigate and accept these mind-body methods as a means of achieving mastery over NAFLD, including them into your everyday practise.

The Role of Exercise in Non Alcoholic Fatty Liver Disease Management

Now that we have discussed the advantages of exercise for NAFLD patients, let's look at how much it can do to improve liver health. The regulation of fat metabolism is one of the many metabolic processes in which the liver is essential. Excess fat builds up in the liver of people with nonalcoholic fatty liver disease (NAFLD), which eventually results in inflammation and damage. Regular exercise, on the other hand, has been demonstrated to counteract this process by enhancing liver function, lowering intrahepatic fat, and stopping further inflammation.

Studies have repeatedly shown that exercise significantly lowers the amount of fat in the liver. Just 12 weeks of moderate-intensity aerobic exercise reduced liver fat in NAFLD patients by an average of 10%, according to a study published in the Journal of Hepatology. This is a significant improvement since it prevents the development of more severe liver disorders including cirrhosis and hepatocellular carcinoma, as well as the progression of the disease.

Exercise is important for liver health, but it's also a critical component of weight control, which is essential for managing nonalcoholic fatty liver disease. The onset and advancement of nonalcoholic fatty liver disease (NAFLD) are closely linked to obesity and excess body weight. Regular physical exercise lowers the risk factors for NAFLD by assisting in the achievement and maintenance of a healthy body weight.

Exercise significantly lowers body weight and body fat percentage in NAFLD patients, according to numerous research. For instance, a 16-week exercise programme including both aerobic and resistance training led to a significant reduction in body weight and body fat percentage in obese NAFLD patients, according to a study published in the European Journal of Sports Science. This underlines how crucial exercise is as a useful tool for addressing the underlying causes of NAFLD and encouraging weight loss.

Exercise can potentially lessen inflammation in NAFLD patients in addition to helping them manage their weight. A defining feature of NAFLD is chronic inflammation, which hastens the course of the illness. It has been demonstrated that exercise has anti-inflammatory properties, inhibiting the release of pro-inflammatory molecules and increasing the synthesis of anti-inflammatory compounds.

Exercise successfully lowers systemic inflammation indicators in people with non-alcoholic fatty liver disease (NAFLD), such as interleukin-6 and C-reactive protein, according to a study published in the journal Obesity Reviews. Exercise has a critical role in controlling inflammation in NAFLD patients, as evidenced by the correlations observed between improvements in insulin sensitivity brought on by exercise and decreases in inflammatory markers.

Exercise has advantages for managing NAFLD that go beyond improving liver health, controlling weight, and reducing inflammation. Frequent physical activity also improves metabolic function, psychological well-being, and cardiovascular fitness, among many other aspects of general health.

Aerobic exercises can enhance cardiovascular fitness and lower the risk of cardiovascular disorders, which are frequently linked to nonalcoholic fatty liver disease (NAFLD). Examples of these exercises include jogging, cycling, swimming, and brisk walking. Exercise also improves glucose utilisation and insulin sensitivity, which lowers the risk of insulin resistance and type 2 diabetes, two conditions that are prevalent comorbidities in non-alcoholic fatty liver disease (NAFLD).

Exercise has also been shown to have psychological advantages and can be a useful coping mechanism for those with non-alcoholic liver disease (NAFLD). It can be emotionally taxing to receive a chronic liver problem diagnosis, which can cause stress, anxiety, and melancholy. Exercise on a regular basis has been demonstrated to increase mood, lessen anxiety and despair, and promote psychological health in general. Exercise produces endorphins, which naturally elevate mood and promote a sense of well-being that helps manage the psychological burden of non-alcoholic fatty liver disease (NAFLD).

Having examined the plethora of advantages exercise provides for individuals with non-alcoholic fatty liver disease (NAFLD), it is imperative to comprehend the pragmatic facets of executing an exercise programme. For best results, a combination of resistance and aerobic activities should be performed.

It is recommended that aerobic exercises, including jogging, cycling, or brisk walking, be done for at least 150 minutes a week, spaced out over multiple days. These exercises raise heart rate, encourage burning of fat, and strengthen the heart. Two to three times a week should be dedicated to resistance activities, such as bodyweight exercises or weightlifting, in order to maintain and increase muscle mass, which is essential for general metabolic health.

Finding an exercise programme that works for each person's tastes and skills is essential because long-term success depends on adherence. People with non-alcoholic fatty liver disease (NAFLD) can incorporate exercise into their daily life by setting reasonable goals, getting expert aid when necessary, and progressively increasing the duration and intensity of their workouts.

In summary, it is impossible to overestimate the importance of exercise in the treatment of nonalcoholic fatty liver disease. Numerous advantages come with exercise, such as better metabolic function, decreased inflammation, weight control, increased cardiovascular fitness, improved liver health, and psychological well-being. People with non-alcoholic fatty liver disease (NAFLD) can take control of their health and strive for the best possible outcomes in their disease management journey by making regular exercise a part of their lives.

Sleep and Non Alcoholic Fatty Liver Disease

Investigating the elements that lead to the onset of the illness is crucial in order to comprehend the relationship between sleep and NAFLD. Fat builds up in the liver, a characteristic of nonalcoholic fatty liver disease (NAFLD) that is not brought on by binge drinking. It frequently coexists with metabolic conditions such insulin resistance, dyslipidemia, and obesity. Sleep disruptions and poor quality of sleep are intimately linked to these metabolic disorders.

The risk of developing non-alcoholic fatty liver disease (NAFLD) is positively correlated with inadequate sleep, according to numerous research investigations. Sleep deprivation can cause abnormalities in the metabolism of fats and carbohydrates, among other metabolic processes. Lack of sleep has been shown to reduce insulin sensitivity, which promotes insulin resistance, a major component in the aetiology of non-alcoholic fatty liver disease. Loss of sleep has also been connected to desires for fatty, high-calorie foods and an increase in appetite, which can lead to weight gain and the buildup of fat in the liver.

Moreover, it has been demonstrated that sleep disruptions encourage oxidative stress and inflammation in the body, two factors that are vital to the development of non-alcoholic fatty liver disease (NAFLD). People who don't get enough sleep are known to have higher levels of inflammatory indicators including interleukin-6 and C-reactive protein. These inflammatory processes raise the likelihood of liver fibrosis and other dangerous consequences, as well as aid in the development and progression of nonalcoholic fatty liver disease (NAFLD).

It is imperative that those who suffer from NAFLD give their sleep hygiene first priority because of the substantial influence that sleep has on the condition. The term "sleep hygiene" describes a collection of attitudes and practises that support restful sleep. I frequently suggest the following methods and techniques to my patients in order to help them sleep better and effectively control their NAFLD:

1. Stick to a consistent sleep schedule: Creating a consistent sleep-wake schedule is crucial for maintaining a healthy internal body clock and encouraging restful sleep. Even on weekends, make an effort to go to bed and wake up at the same time every day.

2. Create a conducive sleep environment: Make sure your bedroom is cold, dark, and quiet. Invest in a comfy pillow and mattress, and get rid of any distractions like electronics or loud noises that can keep you awake.

3. Practice relaxation techniques: Before going to bed, do some relaxing exercises to calm your mind and get your body ready for sleep, including deep breathing, meditation, or light stretching.

4. Limit caffeine and alcohol intake: Alcohol and coffee can both interfere with sleep cycles and reduce the quality of sleep. When it's almost time for bed, steer clear of these and reach for water or herbal teas without caffeine.

5. Establish a bedtime routine: You can tell your body to wind down and get ready for sleep by following a regular pre-sleep regimen. This can involve doing things like curling up with a book, having a warm bath, or listening to relaxing music.

6. Manage stress levels: Stress plays a major role in both NAFLD and sleep problems. Seek out constructive coping strategies to deal with stress, such as mindfulness training or talking to a therapist or support group.

7. Maintain a healthy weight: NAFLD and inadequate sleep quality are closely associated with obesity. Changing to a healthy lifestyle that consists of regular exercise and a nourishing, well-balanced diet can help with weight management as well as sleep patterns.

8. Avoid late-night eating: Eating large meals or heavy snacks right before bed can cause pain and interfere with digestion, making it hard to fall asleep and remain asleep. Try to have your final meal two or three hours before going to bed.

9. Limit screen time before bed: Blue light from electronics like computers, tablets, and cellphones can interfere with the hormone that controls sleep, melatonin production. A minimum of one hour before going to bed, avoid using these devices.

10. Consult with a healthcare professional: After using these tactics, if you still have trouble falling asleep, it could be helpful to consult a healthcare provider. They are able to assess your particular circumstances and offer tailored advice or treatments, including cognitive behavioural therapy for sleeplessness (CBT-I).

By making good sleep hygiene a priority and incorporating these suggestions into your daily routine, you can greatly enhance the quality of your sleep and effectively treat non-alcoholic fatty liver disease (NAFLD). In your quest to conquer non-alcoholic fatty liver disease, keep in mind that sleep is an essential instrument for preserving general health and wellbeing.

Stress Management Techniques

Time Management:

Effective time management is one of the first tactics I advise my patients on. Effective time management enables people to set priorities for their work and devote time to pursuits that improve their physical and emotional health. It lessens the possibility of feeling overwhelmed and fosters a sense of control over one's schedule.

In order to help my patients manage their time effectively, I frequently suggest that they make a daily or weekly calendar. All of their responsibilities, including work or school, family duties, and doctor's appointments, should be included in this calendar. People may then see possible areas for development and have a clear idea of how their time is being used.

I also advise people to make time in their schedules for self-care activities. This covers any kind of relaxation that encourages stress reduction, such as exercise, meditation, or other similar practises. People may make sure they are taking care of their physical and mental health by making time for these activities, which improves stress management.

Relaxation Techniques:

Using relaxation techniques is a crucial component of stress management. By using these methods, people can relax both physically and mentally, which lowers tension and fosters inner peace. Progressive muscle relaxation, guided imagery, and deep breathing exercises are a few well-liked relaxation methods.

During deep breathing exercises, the abdomen should be fully expanded while taking steady, deep breaths. This method is well known for triggering the body's relaxation response, which aids in reducing tension and anxiety in people. Deep breathing exercises are something I frequently recommend to my patients, especially during stressful periods.

The process of progressive muscle relaxation is methodically tensing and relaxing different bodily muscle groups. People feel a general sense of relaxation and are able to release tension from their muscles. This is a strategy that I walk my patients through and urge them to use on a regular basis, either during scheduled relaxation sessions or in stressful situations.

Another effective method of relaxation is guided imagery, which entails utilising visualisation to form serene mental images. When my patients are under stress, I frequently advise them to visualise calm landscapes or listen to guided imagery audios. They can feel more at ease and divert their attention from stressful situations by using this strategy.

Seeking Social Support:

To effectively manage stress, it is essential to seek out social support in addition to time management and relaxation strategies. People can feel validated, understood, and empathetic by talking to others and maintaining a solid support system, which helps lessen the load of stress.

In order to enable my patients to talk about their feelings and experiences dealing with NAFLD, I frequently advise them to get in touch with friends, family, or support groups. This creates a platform for sharing feelings and worries and encourages a sense of community and support.

In addition, partaking in hobbies and pastimes with close friends and family can aid in relaxation and stress relief. People can build healthy relationships, have moments of fun, and ultimately lower their stress levels by engaging in social activities.

If someone does not have a solid support system, I advise getting professional assistance through therapy or counselling. A safe environment to discuss stress-related concerns, acquire coping skills, and create more healthful stress management techniques can be provided by working with a mental health expert.

Conclusion:

To sum up, controlling stress is essential to controlling non-alcoholic fatty liver disease. People can lessen their total stress load by adopting useful practises like time management, relaxation techniques, and reaching out to others for assistance. I advise my patients to prioritise stress management and integrate these strategies into their daily routines as a medical practitioner and health and wellness coach. People with non-alcoholic fatty liver disease can benefit from these initiatives by feeling better overall, having fewer symptoms, and managing their condition more effectively.

The Healing Power of Music and Art

Introduction:

I genuinely believe in the potential of holistic healthcare and wellness as a medical doctor and health and wellness coach. In my experience, treating individuals with Non-Alcoholic Fatty Liver Disease (NAFLD) requires attending to their emotional health in addition to their physical symptoms. We will examine the therapeutic uses of art and music in this chapter to help NAFLD patients feel less stressed and more emotionally well. I will discuss how adding music and art into their lives can improve their general health and well-being using both scientifically supported data and personal tales.

Understanding the Emotional Impact of NAFLD:

For patients, having NAFLD can be emotionally taxing. As people work through the challenges of managing their health, individuals frequently experience a range of feelings, such as worry, depression, and frustration. Emotional distress can also be exacerbated by the physical signs of NAFLD, such as exhaustion and unexplained weight gain or loss.

Stress and Emotional Well-being:

Several investigations have shown a clear connection between stress and the development of NAFLD. In addition to making the disease's symptoms worse, stress raises the possibility of liver damage and inflammation. Thus, addressing stress is crucial for both controlling NAFLD and advancing general health.

The Healing Power of Music:

1. Stress Reduction:

Studies have demonstrated that listening to calming music greatly lowers stress levels. Particularly the soft melodies and harmonies of classical music have been shown in studies to have a relaxing impact on the nervous system, lowering anxiety and fostering relaxation. Stress management can be improved for NAFLD patients by integrating music therapy into their daily routine.

2. Mood Enhancement:

Our emotions can be influenced by music. Uplifting and cheerful music has the power to improve mood and foster happiness and wellbeing. According to studies, listening to music might enhance the release of endorphins, which are inherently uplifting chemicals. NAFLD patients may see an improvement in their emotional health by adding upbeat music to their everyday routines.

3. Pain Management:

For NAFLD patients, pain management is essential, particularly during flare-ups or periods of inflammation. There is ample evidence supporting the use of music in pain treatment. In addition to helping patients feel less pain, listening to music can help release endorphins, which are the body's natural analgesics, and divert attention from their discomfort. NAFLD patients can experience a reduction in the physical discomfort brought on by their condition by participating in music therapy.

The Therapeutic Benefits of Art:

1. Emotional Expression:

Through the medium of art, people may express themselves and share their feelings, ideas, and experiences. Making art can offer NAFLD patients a safe way to express themselves and let go of their emotions, as they frequently struggle to verbalise their emotional issues.

2. Stress Reduction:

It has been demonstrated that making art improves general wellbeing and lowers stress levels. Painting, drawing, or sculpting are examples of creative pursuits that can trigger the body's relaxation response, which lowers blood pressure and heart rate. Patients with non-afflictive learning disabilities (NAFLDs) can reduce stress and find comfort via art therapy.

3. Mindfulness and Meditation:

Making art can be a way to practise meditation and mindfulness. By concentrating on the creative process, people can cultivate a sense of calm and inner peace by being totally present in the moment. Coloring or making mandalas are two art projects that encourage awareness and can help NAFLD patients feel less stressed and more emotionally balanced.

Conclusion:

The emotional and general health of NAFLD patients can be significantly improved by integrating music and art into their daily lives. Music and art therapy can assist a complete approach to controlling non-alcoholic familial liver disease (NAFLD) and supplement conventional medical therapies by lowering stress, improving mood, managing pain, and facilitating emotional expression.

It is my fervent belief as a physician and health and wellness coach that people with NAFLD should investigate the therapeutic benefits of art and music. They can open a door to emotional recovery and well-being by doing creative pursuits, attending art and music therapy classes, or simply listening to and playing their favourite music. NAFLD patients can empower themselves on their path to full NAFLD management by adopting these techniques into their daily life.

The Importance of Emotional Well-being

Handling a chronic illness such as non-alcoholic fatty liver disease (NAFLD) can be difficult since it frequently necessitates major lifestyle changes and the adoption of new routines. Negative feelings like irritation, worry, and even despair can result from these drastic and unpleasant shifts. But we can improve our capacity to effectively manage NAFLD and, in the end, live healthier lives if we place a higher priority on our emotional well-being.

According to research, controlling chronic illnesses, such as NAFLD, requires a strong emotional foundation. In the Journal of Psychosomatic Research, for example, a study indicated that better disease management outcomes were achieved by NAFLD patients who reported higher levels of psychological well-being. These results imply that we can better follow treatment regimens, make healthier decisions, and attain better health outcomes when we are emotionally stable.

Because it lowers stress and encourages healthy lifestyle changes, keeping an optimistic outlook is crucial to managing non-alcoholic fatty liver disease (NAFLD). Positivity and optimism about our condition increase our likelihood of doing things like regular exercise and eating a balanced diet that can help our livers function better. Furthermore, as stress is believed to hasten the development of NAFLD, having a positive outlook helps us create coping mechanisms that may efficiently manage and lessen it.

Developing a self-care mindset is one of the cornerstones of preserving emotional health. Setting our physical, mental, and emotional needs first is a key component of self-care. It's a comprehensive method that includes a variety of tactics and endeavours to advance general health. Activities that lower stress, such mindfulness meditation or creative hobbies, might be considered self-care in the context of non-alcoholic fatty liver disease (NAFLD).

Our emotional health can be greatly impacted by asking for help from others in addition to practising self-care. Compared to other chronic disorders, NAFLD is not as well-known or understood, which can make it feel lonely. However, making connections with people who have gone through comparable things can offer validation and a sense of community. For those with non-alcoholic fatty liver disease (NAFLD), support groups and online forums can be very helpful since they provide a safe environment for sharing struggles and achievements.

Psychiatric methods and counselling can also be quite helpful in regulating emotional health. We can investigate and treat any underlying emotional problems or mental health issues that might be affecting our capacity to properly manage NAFLD by working with a counsellor or therapist. Additionally, therapy can support the development of constructive thought patterns and coping mechanisms that foster emotional resilience.

An additional facet of emotional well-being that warrants consideration is the correlation between mental health and nutrition. Several research have demonstrated a reciprocal association between nutrition and mental health, with unhealthy eating habits raising the chance of mental health issues and mental health conditions causing disordered eating behaviours. As a result, it is critical to give equal weight to a nutritious, balanced diet for both mental and hepatic health.

Though it may not always be simple, there are clear advantages to using techniques to preserve mental stability and a positive outlook when managing non-alcoholic fatty liver disease (NAFLD). As evidenced by research, people with better emotional health and a happy outlook on life are actually more likely to sustain healthy lifestyle choices and see improvements in their NAFLD outcomes.

Gratitude and mindfulness exercises are beneficial for developing a happy outlook. Even though treating NAFLD can be difficult, these techniques can help us focus on the here and now and cultivate gratitude for the positive aspects of our lives. Regular physical activity has also been demonstrated to improve mood and lower stress levels, which improves emotional well-being.

In summary, the management of non-alcoholic fatty liver disease necessitates putting emotional well-being first and keeping an optimistic outlook. Effective management of non-alcoholic fatty liver disease (NAFLD) can be improved by acknowledging the influence of emotional state on health outcomes and using methods to promote emotional well-being. In the context of NAFLD, there are many strategies and techniques available to improve mental well-being, ranging from self-care routines to counselling and asking for help. Recall that in addition to healing our liver, we are also fostering our mental health in order to advance general well-being.

Chapter 6: Customizable Plans for Non Alcoholic Fatty Liver Disease Management

Personalized Diet Plans

Prior to creating a customised diet plan, it is essential to comprehend the underlying causes of a person's non-alcoholic fatty liver disease (NAFLD). Numerous factors come into play, including age, gender, body composition, metabolic health, and way of life. By compiling this data, we can design a strategy that takes into account the particular requirements of every patient and aids in the achievement of their health objectives.

First, we perform a comprehensive evaluation of the person's present eating patterns and way of life. This entails assessing their calorie intake each day, the distribution of macronutrients, nutritional inadequacies, and food preferences. Knowing their baseline diet enables us to pinpoint areas for improvement and create a patient-friendly, long-lasting plan.

We also consider the patient's desired state of health. Some people could put weight loss first, while others might concentrate on lowering inflammation or enhancing liver function. We can provide the patient with better assistance on their path to optimal liver health if the food plan is in line with these objectives.

When designing the personalized diet plan, we consider the following key principles:

1. Balanced Macronutrient Distribution: For general health and liver function, a balanced intake of macronutrients—carbs, proteins, and fats—is necessary. In close collaboration with patients, we ascertain the ideal macronutrient ratio based on each person's unique requirements and objectives.

2. Emphasis on Whole Foods: Consuming a diet high in whole, unprocessed foods reduces exposure to harmful chemicals and preservatives while also supplying vital nutrients. We assist patients in adding whole grains, fruits, vegetables, lean meats, and healthy fats to their regular diets.

3. Portion Control: For the purpose of limiting calorie intake and reaching weight loss objectives, portion control is essential. We give patients advice on appropriate serving sizes and useful techniques to assist them in controlling their portion sizes.

4. Avoidance of High Glycemic Index Foods: High glycemic index foods may exacerbate NAFLD by spiking blood sugar levels. In order to help patients maintain healthy liver function and regulate blood sugar levels, we inform them about the glycemic index and suggest low-GI diets.

5. Customized Meal Plans: We design individualised meal plans based on the patient's dietary requirements, lifestyle, and cultural background to guarantee long-term compliance and success. This method considers individual tastes, which increases the diet's sustainability and enjoyment.

6. Monitoring Progress: It's critical to do routine monitoring and follow-ups in order to assess development, make required modifications, and offer continuous assistance. We advise patients to record their food consumption in a food diary so that we can monitor it and make any necessary adjustments.

7. Collaboration with Other Health Professionals: We work in tandem with other medical specialists, including certified nutritionists, psychologists, and fitness trainers, as part of the all-encompassing approach to managing non-alcoholic fast-living disorders. Through these partnerships, patients are guaranteed to receive comprehensive care that attends to both their physical and mental needs.

Personalized diet programmes involve more than just limiting your intake of specific foods or adhering to a predetermined format. They are intended to provide people the power to alter their lifestyles in a way that will improve the health of their livers. We can assist individuals with NAFLD in efficiently managing their illness by customising diet regimens to meet their unique needs, preferences, and health objectives.

To sum up, customised eating regimens are essential for managing nonalcoholic fatty liver disease. We may design a plan that is specific to the needs, preferences, and health objectives of each individual by evaluating them. We offer complete care to NAFLD patients by distributing macronutrients in a balanced way, emphasising whole foods, controlling portions, avoiding foods with a high glycemic index, creating personalised meal plans, keeping track of progress, and working with other medical specialists. I firmly think that people with non-alcoholic fatty liver disease (NAFLD) may take charge of their health and achieve better liver function with the correct support and individualised care.

Exercise and Fitness Plans

It's crucial to first determine each patient's degree of fitness. This can be achieved by putting them through a battery of physical examinations and tests, like ones that gauge their flexibility, strength, and cardiovascular endurance. These evaluations will assist me in figuring out the patient's initial level of fitness and pointing out any areas that require development.

After getting all the information I need, I can create a customised workout programme for every patient. This plan will include their level of fitness at the moment, any potential physical restrictions, and their preferred workout regimens. The benefits of exercise can be maximised while the risk of discomfort or injury is reduced by designing a personalised regimen.

I frequently begin low-impact workouts like walking or swimming with patients who have substantial physical restrictions or poor fitness levels. These exercises are easy to adapt to the capacities of the individual and are mild on the joints. Especially walking, which can be customised to varying intensities and durations based on the patient's demands, is an excellent means of increasing cardiovascular endurance.

I can progressively add more difficult workouts to the patient's regimen as their level of fitness increases and their physical restrictions lessen. Exercises like weight training, cycling, and mild running may fall under this category. Patients with non-alcoholic fatty liver disease can benefit most from strength training since it can aid with insulin sensitivity and muscle mass.

I advise my patients to include mobility and flexibility exercises in their routine in addition to strength and cardiovascular activities. These exercises facilitate greater range of motion in the joints, lessen stiffness in the muscles, and improve general physical function. Stretching, yoga, and Pilates are examples of activities that can be tailored to each patient's unique needs.

Regularly tracking my patients' development is crucial to ensuring the efficacy of the fitness regimen. Physical evaluations, frequent check-ins, and monitoring of their workout logs can all help achieve this. I may continue to challenge the patient while maintaining their safety and comfort by keeping an eye on their development and making any required adjustments to the workout regimen.

For individuals with non-alcoholic fatty liver disease, exercise has many psychological and emotional advantages in addition to its physical ones. Frequent exercise promotes general wellbeing, happiness, and a reduction in stress. In addition, it can function as a constructive coping mechanism for handling the difficulties and pressures linked to this illness.

To help my patients stay motivated and dedicated to their fitness goals, I not only provide them training regimens but also advice and encouragement. This covers instruction on the advantages of consistent exercise, advice on getting beyond fitness obstacles, and methods for keeping an active lifestyle. In order to maximise the possibility of long-term adherence to the fitness plan, I also advise my patients to discover hobbies and activities that fit into their lifestyle.

Finally, a key element of my all-encompassing strategy for treating nonalcoholic fatty liver disease is providing individualised fitness and exercise regimens to patients. Maximizing the advantages of exercise while lowering the risk of discomfort or injury is possible when I customise the exercise plan to the individual's fitness level, restrictions, and preferences. Frequent exercise enhances mental and emotional well-being in addition to physical health. I work to assist my patients in reaching their fitness objectives and enhancing their general well-being by offering direction, support, and frequent monitoring.

Stress Management Plans

Everybody reacts to stress in a different way, so what suits one person may not suit another. For this reason, I think it's important to help my patients develop stress-reduction strategies that include methods specific to their own interests and way of life. By doing this, individuals have a higher chance of incorporating these habits into their daily lives and maintaining them, which will improve their general health and liver function.

I take the time to learn about the client's lifestyle, daily schedule, and particular stressors during the first consultation. This aids me in determining the best stress-reduction strategies for them. I also take into account any current health issues or drugs they are taking because certain stress-reduction strategies may interact with these things.

I usually suggest a variety of stress-reduction strategies to my NAFLD patients. These methods may be advantageous for liver health in addition to lowering stress. I go over each technique with the patient, outlining its advantages and practical applications.

I frequently suggest mindfulness meditation as one method. Regular mindfulness meditation practise lowers stress and enhances emotional well-being, according to research. Patients can reduce stress and improve the health of their livers by focusing on the here and now and letting go of their problems. I encourage my patients to practise mindfulness for a few minutes every day by teaching them various techniques including body scanning and breath awareness.

Exercise is another method for stress management that I think is helpful. Endorphins are naturally occurring hormones that are released when you exercise. Frequent exercise helps regulate weight and improve insulin sensitivity, two important aspects of maintaining non-alcoholic fatty liver disease (NAFLD). It also reduces stress. Together, my patients and I create an exercise programme that works for their tastes and degree of fitness. This can involve exercises like cycling, yoga, swimming, or brisk walking.

I also stress the value of a balanced diet in reducing stress and enhancing liver health, in addition to mindfulness and exercise. It has been discovered that some foods, such as those rich in omega-3 fatty acids, vitamin C, and magnesium, have a beneficial effect on stress levels. Together with a dietitian, I create customised meal programmes that include these calming foods. Patients can support the health of their livers in addition to managing their stress levels by giving their bodies the correct nutrients.

Long-term NAFLD management requires integrating stress-relieving activities into daily living. I provide my patients tools and support to help them put these strategies into practise. This could be giving them pointers about apps for relaxation or recordings of guided meditation, telling them about fitness centres or support groups in the area, or putting them in touch with other health care providers, like acupuncturists or therapists, who can provide more stress-reduction resources.

In addition, I advise my patients to undertake self-care methods that they find meaningful. This can entail taking up enjoyable hobbies, going outside, or doing deep breathing techniques. Finding things that they enjoy doing and that help them decompress from the stresses of everyday life is the aim.

Plans for stress management must also include coping mechanisms. I collaborate closely with my patients to create coping strategies that help them manage stressors. This could entail learning how to set limits, improving problem-solving abilities, or reframing negative ideas with encouraging statements. By providing my patients with these resources, they can manage stressful situations more skillfully and preserve the health of their livers.

Lastly, I underline the significance of routine self-evaluation and strategy modification for stress management. Stress levels fluctuate, so what worked at first might not work as well later. I advise my patients to frequently assess their stress levels and make any adjustments to their stress-reduction strategy. This guarantees that their current stress-reduction methods remain efficient and encourages a proactive attitude to stress management.

In summary, helping patients with non-alcoholic fatty liver disease develop individualised stress management strategies is an essential part of their total care. Patients are more likely to embrace and maintain these practises when they incorporate strategies that align with their lifestyle and preferences, which can improve liver health and overall well-being. Patients can effectively manage their stress and maintain long-term liver health by combining self-care, exercise, a good diet, mindfulness, and coping skills. It is an honour for me to provide my patients with the skills and information necessary to successfully and confidently traverse their NAFLD journey.

Sleep Improvement Plans

A vital component of human health, sleep affects several physiological functions, including the health of our livers. Numerous studies have demonstrated a direct link between low-quality sleep and the onset and development of non-alcoholic fatty liver disease (NAFLD). Increased liver inflammation, insulin resistance, and hepatic fat buildup can result from sleep disruptions that are common in people with nonalcoholic fatty liver disease (NAFLD), including sleep apnea, insomnia, and restless legs syndrome.

I use an all-encompassing strategy that blends evidence-based techniques with individualised plans made to meet each patient's unique needs in order to address these problems and assist patients in improving the quality of their sleep. Prior to delving into the tactics and methods, it's critical to comprehend the causes of insomnia and how they affect non-alcoholic fatty liver disease.

Anxiety and stress are frequent causes of sleep problems, and NAFLD patients frequently have higher stress levels because of the difficulty of controlling their condition. Furthermore, insufficient sleep can worsen worry and stress, starting a vicious cycle that endangers the functioning of the liver. Thus, stress-reduction methods like mindfulness meditation, yoga, and counselling are essential parts of any sleep-improvement strategy.

Our internal biological clock, known as the circadian rhythm, which controls sleep-wake cycles, is another important element influencing the quality of our sleep. Sleep problems and an elevated risk of non-alcoholic fatty liver disease (NAFLD) have been associated with circadian rhythm disruptions. I suggest establishing a regular sleep pattern, avoiding bright lights—especially blue light from electronics—before bed, and developing a calming nighttime ritual to tell the body it's time to wind down in order to maximise the circadian rhythm.

Improving the quality of sleep also requires creating a comfortable sleeping environment. A quiet, cool, and dark bedroom encourages restful, deep sleep. In order to establish a tranquil sleep sanctuary, I frequently counsel patients to purchase blackout curtains, earplugs, white noise machines, and cosy bedding. Furthermore, using relaxation methods before bed to help the body enter a peaceful sleep-promoting state, such as deep breathing exercises or light stretching, can be beneficial.

Healthy sleep is greatly aided by diet, and for those with non-alcoholic fatty liver disease (NAFLD), diet becomes even more important. Healthy fats, lean protein, and fiber-rich foods can help control blood sugar levels and minimise swings that could interfere with sleep. Furthermore, dietary modifications are crucial for better sleep quality in NAFLD patients because stimulants like caffeine and alcohol can disrupt sleep patterns.

Frequent exercise helps to improve the quality of sleep in addition to its benefits for liver function. Deeper, more peaceful sleep can be encouraged by participating in moderate-intensity exercise, such yoga or brisk walking, for at least half an hour most days of the week. This will help balance the sleep-wake cycle. But, it's crucial to steer clear of strenuous exercise right before bed because it can have a stimulating effect and make it more difficult to fall asleep.

Apart from these broad approaches, I collaborate extensively with every patient to develop customised sleep enhancement programmes that are suited to their individual requirements and situations. This can entail locating and treating any underlying sleep disorders—like restless leg syndrome or sleep apnea—by directing them to sleep specialists. On an individual basis, combining evidence-based methods with complementary techniques like acupuncture, herbal supplements, or aromatherapy may also be taken into consideration.

For those with non-alcoholic fatty liver disease (NAFLD), cognitive-behavioral treatment for insomnia (CBT-I) is a useful strategy that can be included in sleep improvement regimens. Without the risks and adverse effects of sleep drugs, cognitive behavioural therapy (CBT-I) has been shown to be just as effective as, if not more so, in treating the beliefs and behaviours that lead to insomnia.

In summary, improving sleep quality is essential to successfully controlling non-alcoholic fatty liver disease (NAFLD). Patients can take proactive steps to improve the quality of their sleep, improve liver health, and improve their general well-being by receiving useful strategies and individualised sleep improvement plans. We can enable patients with nonalcoholic fatty liver disease (NAFLD) to take charge of their sleep and, ultimately, their liver health by using a comprehensive approach that takes into account a variety of factors that impact sleep, including stress, circadian rhythm disruption, sleep environment, food, and physical activity. Never forget that achieving appropriate sleep quality and improving NAFLD management can be achieved with minor tweaks and persistent effort.

Holistic Wellness Plans

As a physician and wellness and health coach, I am a strong proponent of holistic medicine. Adopting holistic wellness techniques has proven beneficial for numerous individuals with Non Alcoholic Fatty Liver Disease (NAFLD) that I have observed in my clinic. Self-care, self-reflection, and mindfulness are among of the techniques that can help manage NAFLD and enhance general wellbeing.

It's critical to change the emphasis of NAFLD management from merely treating the disease's outward symptoms to addressing its underlying causes and fostering liver health in general. Plans for holistic wellbeing provide a multifaceted approach that considers the physical, mental, and emotional well-being of the individual.

For NAFLD patients, developing a comprehensive health strategy requires mindfulness. People who practise mindfulness might become more conscious of their thoughts, feelings, and body. This knowledge can assist them in determining possible NAFLD symptom triggers, such as stress or unhealthful eating patterns. To assist patients in developing this awareness, I frequently lead them through mindfulness exercises in my practise, like body scans and deep breathing.

Another essential component of a comprehensive wellness programme for NAFLD patients is self-care. It entails making a conscious decision to put one's physical and emotional health first. Self-care strategies for NAFLD patients can include maintaining a balanced diet, exercising frequently, getting enough sleep, and learning stress reduction methods. These self-care techniques enhance general wellness in addition to liver function.

For NAFLD patients, developing customised wellness programmes entails taking into account their particular requirements, objectives, and preferences. In my practise, I collaborate extensively with every patient to create a personalised strategy that addresses their unique circumstances. This entails evaluating their food preferences, degree of exercise, stress level, and any other elements that might have an effect on the health of their liver. I also consider lifestyle considerations while making recommendations, making sure they are doable and sustainable for them.

Personalized wellness plans for people with non-alcoholic fatty liver disease (NAFLD) include nutritional counselling. According to research, some foods can make NAFLD symptoms worse while others are good for the liver. I can assist each patient in making decisions that support liver health by thoroughly examining their diet and providing tailored advice. This could entail increasing the intake of fruits, vegetables, whole grains, lean proteins, and lowering or eliminating items high in added sugars, processed carbs, and saturated fats.

Another crucial element of a comprehensive wellness programme for NAFLD patients is exercise. Frequent exercise has been demonstrated to enhance general health, lower inflammation, and enhance liver function. Nonetheless, it's critical to consider the unique level of fitness and any potential physical restrictions of each patient. In my practise, I collaborate with patients to create a safe, capacity-appropriate fitness programme. Combinations of cardiovascular, strength, and flexibility training may be part of this.

For individuals with NAFLD, stress management is also essential to a comprehensive wellness programme. Prolonged stress can worsen symptoms and has been related to the development of NAFLD. Patients can lower their stress levels and improve the health of their livers by implementing stress management practises into their everyday routine. These methods could include breathing exercises, relaxing methods, and identifying constructive ways to decompress, including hobbies or time spent in nature.

In addition to stress reduction, self-care, and mindfulness, self-reflection is a crucial technique that can help NAFLD patients on their path to better health. Taking the time to consider one's ideas, emotions, and actions while recognising opportunities for development and constructive change is known as self-reflection. In my work, I frequently lead patients through self-reflection activities to help them understand their own health and wellbeing, such as journaling or guided visualisation.

I have seen amazing gains in the health and well-being of NAFLD patients by encouraging them to embrace holistic wellness practises and helping them create customised wellness regimens. Plans for holistic wellness offer a whole approach to managing non-alcoholic fatty liver disease (NAFLD), addressing not just the disease's clinical symptoms but also its underlying causes and emotional elements. NAFLD sufferers can regain their health and have active, satisfying lives by adopting a comprehensive approach.

Monitoring and Tracking Progress

Why is progress tracking and monitoring so important in the management of NAFLD? The explanation for this is that non-alcoholic fatty liver disease (NAFLD) is a multifactorial illness. Genetics, way of life decisions, eating patterns, and general health are some of these variables. Because of this, each person responds to treatment regimens differently in terms of their efficacy. We are able to determine what is most effective for each patient and modify treatment approaches by routinely observing and recording progress.

Evaluating the effects of lifestyle changes on liver health objectively is one of the main advantages of tracking and monitoring progress. It has been demonstrated that modifying one's lifestyle to include more physical activity and nutritional alterations can help with non-alcoholic fatty liver disease. Through monitoring alterations in liver enzyme levels, lipid composition, and general liver function, we can ascertain whether these lifestyle changes are actually advantageous for a certain patient.

I frequently suggest routine blood tests to evaluate liver enzymes, such as alanine aminotransferase (ALT) and aspartate aminotransferase, in order to assist patients in keeping an eye on the condition of their livers (AST). Increased concentrations of these enzymes are suggestive of injury and inflammation in the liver. Patients can track the efficacy of their treatment programmes and make appropriate modifications by routinely evaluating these levels.

Apart from liver enzymes, specialist imaging methods like transient elastography and magnetic resonance imaging (MRI) can also evaluate other indicators of liver function, like liver fat content and fibrosis. These techniques offer a more thorough picture of a patient's liver health and can direct therapy choices.

Moreover, progress tracking and monitoring go beyond liver health. The metabolic syndrome, which encompasses diseases including obesity, high blood pressure, and raised blood sugar, is intimately linked to non-alcoholic fatty liver disease (NAFLD). We can follow gains in general metabolic health in addition to identifying underlying risk factors for NAFLD with regular monitoring of these measures.

In the current digital era, there are many tools and resources available for monitoring many facets of health and well-being. Apps for smartphones can be a terrific way to easily track medication adherence, physical activity levels, and eating habits. Tracking blood pressure, blood sugar, weight, and other pertinent health markers is another feature that many applications provide. By identifying patterns and trends, this data can offer important insights into the efficacy of therapeutic measures and lifestyle changes.

Wearable technology has become more and more popular in recent years, including fitness trackers and smartwatches, in addition to smartphone apps. These gadgets can monitor stress levels, heart rates, sleep patterns, and even steps. A more complete picture of general health and well-being can be acquired by combining data from these devices with other health markers, such as liver enzymes and metabolic parameters.

Although technology has made tracking and monitoring progress easier than ever, it's crucial to avoid becoming unduly dependent on these resources. A key component of attentive monitoring is self-awareness and mindfulness. It is important for patients to constantly try to be aware of their bodies and record any changes or symptoms that could need more care.

Moreover, measuring and monitoring development shouldn't be limited to physical well-being. The psychological and emotional health of NAFLD patients is just as vital. It can be difficult mentally to manage a chronic illness, so it's important to take care of any emotional or psychological issues that may come up.

Support groups, counselling, and therapy can give patients a secure setting in which to talk about their experiences and look for advice. I frequently use coping mechanisms and psychology-related approaches in my therapy to assist patients in stress management and upholding an optimistic outlook throughout their NAFLD journey.

All things considered, tracking and monitoring development is a crucial component of NAFLD management. It enables us to determine what needs to be improved, make the required modifications, and impartially evaluate the efficacy of therapy interventions. Patients can actively engage in their own care and take charge of their health and well-being by making use of the tools and resources accessible to them in the current digital era. Don't undervalue the importance of keeping an eye on your development; it may hold the secret to effectively managing nonalcoholic fatty liver disease (NAFLD) and attaining ideal liver health.

Adjusting Plans as Needed

I always begin developing a NAFLD management strategy by stressing how important it is to make lifestyle changes. This include taking up a balanced diet, getting more exercise, and controlling stress. Any NAFLD management plan must start with these lifestyle adjustments, but it's important to understand that each person will react differently to them. Since every person's path to liver recovery is different, it is our duty as medical professionals to support them in making the required modifications in light of their development and evolving situation.

Monitoring Progress

First and foremost, it's critical to consistently assess our patients' progress. This include doing liver imaging studies, evaluating blood lipid profiles, and routinely testing their liver enzymes. These objective metrics offer insightful information on the effectiveness of their present strategy and assist in identifying any areas that might need modification. Patients must be made aware of the importance of these tests and assisted in understanding how to interpret the results.

These findings allow us to pinpoint areas in need of additional focus. For instance, it can be essential to reevaluate a patient's activity level or look into alternative physical activities that would be more beneficial for them if their liver enzymes are still elevated even after they have just begun a new exercise programme. Similarly, dietary or medication changes may be necessary if their blood lipid profile shows consistently elevated cholesterol levels.

Regular Communication

For us to make necessary adjustments to programmes, constant communication with our patients is just as important as objective measurements. It's critical to establish a space where kids feel at ease discussing their worries, challenges, and victories. We can better comprehend their experiences by having honest and open discussions, which enables us to provide the right advice and assistance.

It is imperative that we, as healthcare providers, take a patient-centered approach and pay close attention to their input. Individuals could have physical changes that are not immediately detected by laboratory testing. For example, after implementing specific dietary adjustments, a patient might report feeling more energised or having improved digestion. We should never discount these subjective feelings because they offer important information about the patient's general health and can help us make the required corrections.

Tailoring Diet and Nutrition

When it comes to managing non-alcoholic fatty liver disease (NAFLD), diet and nutrition are crucial and frequently call for the biggest changes. Although broad dietary guidelines can serve as a foundation, it is crucial to customise these suggestions according to personal requirements and inclinations. This could entail working with a dietician or nutritionist to create a customised meal plan that takes the patient's lifestyle and cultural background into account.

Patients may go through weight fluctuations, metabolic profile alterations, or new dietary limitations as a result of other medical issues along the NAFLD management journey. It could be necessary to make adjustments to account for these changes. For instance, a patient who at first fared well on a low-carb diet might discover that, in order to maintain their energy levels or fulfil the demands of their exercise programme, they must consume more carbohydrates.

Psychological and Emotional Considerations

Managing non-alcoholic fatty liver disease (NAFLD) entails not only addressing physical abnormalities but also psychological and emotional issues. People with NAFLD frequently experience feelings of frustration, remorse, and shame. They could struggle to follow through on their intentions or run into obstacles along the road. It is imperative that we as medical professionals give our patients the support and direction they need to deal with these feelings.

Plans may need to be adjusted to accommodate psychological and emotional requirements, which may entail adding counselling or therapy sessions to the overall plan of care. These sessions can assist people in strengthening their resilience, creating coping mechanisms, and addressing any underlying psychological issues that might be impeding their development. We can provide our patients the tools they need to make the required changes and take back control of their health by taking care of these issues.

Coping with Changing Circumstances

In addition to taking individual growth into account, modifying plans as necessary also entails reacting to a patient's evolving circumstances. Since life is unpredictable, our plans need to be adaptable enough to take these unforeseen events into account. For instance, a stressful incident like losing their job or losing a loved one may cause a patient to have a brief setback. It could be required to give them more assistance and direction during these periods, as well as to review their management plan to make sure it still applies to their present situation.

In a similar vein, patients' objectives may change as they move forward with the care of their NAFLD. At first, lowering liver enzymes and enhancing metabolic indicators might be the main priorities. But as these objectives are met, attention might turn to preserving liver health over the long term and stopping the disease's progression. It could be necessary to make changes to the management plan to account for these evolving objectives.

The Power of Self-care and Alternative Techniques

Apart from conventional medical interventions, alternative approaches and self-care can be effective strategies in the management of non-alcoholic fatty liver disease (NAFLD). These methods, which include yoga, acupuncture, herbal medicine, and mindfulness exercises, can support patients further and supplement traditional therapies. People may discover great advantages in adding these methods to their current management plans, depending on their interests and preferences.

It is our duty as healthcare providers to tell patients about these alternatives and assist them in making defensible choices. Many people find that these practises are beneficial for stress management, relaxation, and enhancing general well-being, even though the evidence supporting some of them may be weak. In the end, the goal is to give patients the confidence to take charge of their health and experiment with methods that work for them.

Conclusion

To sum up, emphasising the necessity of adaptation and flexibility in NAFLD treatment regimens is essential for enabling patients to take charge of their own liver repair. It can be necessary to make adjustments in light of each person's development, evolving conditions, and evolving objectives. We can offer our patients complete assistance by keeping track of their development, staying in constant contact, customising diet and nutrition, attending to psychological and emotional issues, and combining self-care and alternative methods. In the end, we can assist people in achieving total non-alcoholic fatty liver disease treatment and enhance their general health by working together.

Celebrating Milestones and Achievements

Let's first examine the definition of a milestone in the context of NAFLD management before moving on to discuss the importance of recognising and celebrating them. Anything, no matter how minor, that indicates advancement on our path to a healthier liver should be considered a milestone. It could be hitting a particular weight loss target, sticking to a balanced diet for a predetermined amount of time, getting regular exercise, or even getting better findings from a liver health examination. Every person has several milestones that vary based on their specific objectives and aspirations.

We must recognise the enormous obstacles that people with NAFLD confront in order to fully appreciate the significance of commemorating these accomplishments. A major lifestyle makeover, including adjustments to food, exercise regimen, and general outlook on health and wellbeing, is necessary to manage this illness. Maintaining these improvements and staying on course requires an enormous amount of discipline, commitment, and willpower.

It is all too easy to lose motivation and feel discouraged during this difficult road, especially if results take a while to show. For this reason, a key element of our NAFLD management plan is marking milestones. We may improve our mood, increase our sense of self-worth, and reaffirm our resolve to live a healthier lifestyle by taking the time to recognise and celebrate our successes.

There are many different ways to treat oneself after accomplishing a goal; in the end, the decision comes down to what makes each person happy and fulfilled. Here are some ideas to think about:

1. Pamper Yourself: Give yourself a massage, a spa day, or a soothing bath using essential oils. Throughout this journey, it is imperative that

we take care of our physical and emotional health. A little self-care can go a long way toward reviving our motivation and spirit.

2. Indulge in a Healthy Feast: Celebrate your success with a special dinner that is made using wholesome ingredients. This may be a trip to your preferred health-conscious restaurant or a cooked gourmet meal. Savoring each bite satisfies your palate while also commemorating your accomplishments.

3. Engage in a Hobby: Spend some time engaging in a hobby or pastime that makes you happy and helps you unwind. Painting, dancing, gardening, or any other activity that piques your interest could be it. Partaking in these pursuits not only fosters your artistic side but also relieves tension.

4. Plan a Social Gathering: Throw a celebration for your milestone and invite friends and family. It may be a virtual get-together, a picnic, or a modest dinner party. Being surrounded by people you love and telling them about your accomplishments fosters a sense of support, encouragement, and community.

5. Document Your Progress: Maintain a visual log of your accomplishments and benchmarks. This could be an electronic folder, a scrapbook, or a notebook. You can appreciate the transforming journey you are on and look back on how far you have come by keeping a record of your progress.

6. Invest in Education: Think about signing up for a workshop, seminar, or course that fits your objectives and areas of interest. Increasing your knowledge gives you the information and resources you need to continue on your path to ideal liver health while also rewarding your hard work.

7. Upgrade Your Wardrobe: Give yourself a new look or accessory that boosts your self-esteem and makes you feel good about your achievements. It's critical to accept our new selves and acknowledge the improvements we've made as our bodies evolve.

Recall that the rewards you choose should be based on your own interests and preferences; these are just ideas. The goal is to recognise and honour your diligence, commitment, and advancement toward NAFLD management.

By emphasising the celebration of life events and accomplishments, we establish a positive feedback loop that inspires us to keep choosing better decisions. This celebration not only serves as a reminder of our accomplishments but also fosters the growth of a resilient mindset that will help us overcome any obstacles in our path.

In summary, acknowledging and appreciating accomplishments is critical to the treatment of nonalcoholic fatty liver disease. It gives us the much-needed inspiration and drive to press on with our quest for a healthier liver and a higher standard of living. Therefore, my dear readers, I urge you to take the time to recognise and celebrate each milestone—no matter how small—as you set out on this life-changing adventure. Never forget that every step you take is a step in the right direction, and you should be honoured for your devotion and hard work.

Milton Keynes UK
Ingram Content Group UK Ltd.
UKHW020645120124
435917UK00015B/516